*Cindy Says®...*

# "You Can Find Health in Your Hectic World"

## Healthy Lifestyle Advice

### By Cindy Boggs

Copyright © 2007 **Cindy Boggs**
*All Rights Reserved*

*CindySays*® is a registered trademark

First Edition

Published by The Printing Press Ltd.
Charleston, West Virginia

Cover Design and Illustrations
Jeff Pierson

Photos
Steve Payne Photography

Layout Design Coordinator
Jeff Beary

Editor
Jim Wallace

ISBN: 978-0-9791345-0-0

# Dedication

To my grandson Tino, who reminds me each day that he's forming his lifestyle habits by watching ours.

# Acknowledgements

*This book found its way here with a little coaxing and a great deal of support from those around me. I am grateful for their presence in my life and their unique assistance.*

To my father, who instilled in me the desire to care about the well-being of others; to my son, Craig, who first conceived of and strongly suggested I tackle this project; to my sons, Jeff, for his artistic eye; Rocky for his business sense, and daughters-in-law, Apryll and Cherilyn, who have been dependable sources of encouragement throughout the process; and to my talented sister, Debbie, for her ability to make the difficult seem easy and for being my greatest advisor.

A sincere expression of thanks goes to Craig Selby, who first saw merit in my writing and offered me the opportunity to create a health and fitness column for the Charleston Newspapers; to Doug Imbrogno, the catalyst responsible for a significant change of direction in my life, who consistently dreams big for me; and to Rosalie Earle who allows me freedom to experiment with my writing.

I'm reasonably sure this book couldn't have been written without the support of the Charleston YMCA. For 18 years, the YMCA has been my training ground and my point of contact with the people represented in this book. I want to especially thank Jesse Madden and Greg Cottrill for trusting me to fulfill my duties as fitness coordinator while giving me the necessary daytime hours to devote to writing. Also, the process wouldn't have been nearly as exciting without the frequent motivation I received from John Giroir and Rebecca Loughry—their confidence in me was remarkably inspiring.

I am eternally grateful for the insight gained from my readers, who are responsible for the subject matter and continue to supply me and challenge me with wonderfully provocative questions for my CindySays column. To Nancy Braenovich, Patti Carnemolla, Susan Gentilin, Lyne Ranson and Cathy Capps-Amburgey, who offered everything from legal advice to comic relief.

To my writing group, Laurie Helgoe, Bruce Haley, Jim Wallace and Beth Wheatley, who lend attention, affection and direction to this sometimes-overwhelming experience and who remind me to see the joy of the process; a special thank-you to Jim for his meticulous editing skills and willingness to read every word.

To Dr. Wayne Westcott, whose trusted research has fed my curiosity, facilitated my work and inspired me to share my advice with others; to Strongest Man in the World, Phil Pfister, whose accomplishments remind us that the proud men, women and children of West Virginia have immeasurable strength.

Finally, as a citizen of West Virginia interested in health, I am exceptionally proud to be working on issues of obesity while serving on the Healthy Lifestyle Coalition under the direction of our First Lady, Gayle Manchin. The First Lady is directly linked to the positive changes in West Virginia's state of health. She guides us with a genuine determination for measurable health improvements and inspires us with her level of commitment and dedicated focus toward Governor Manchin's health initiatives.

The Governor and First Lady's support is an amazing gift. I thank them for their consistent leadership on a matter that is at the heart of every West Virginian.

# Foreword

As governor of West Virginia, I am blessed in being able to lead one of the most beautiful states in the nation. But I am dedicated to making it a better place to live, and this includes improving the health of our people. Like many Americans, we have fallen into sedentary lifestyles with too much food and not enough nutrition. That is why First Lady Gayle Manchin and I are working to promote exercise, proper diet and other aspects of a healthy lifestyle.

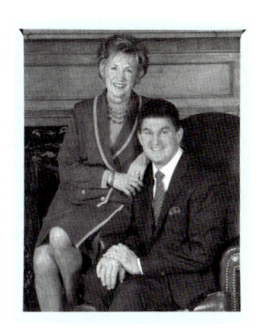

We recognize that government policy can be a catalyst, but personal accountability is at the heart of adopting long-term healthy habits. Furthermore, while the support of family and friends is important, each individual must take responsibility for his or her own health. However, it can be a daunting task to figure out how to achieve the right mix of physical activity and nutritious foods while avoiding fads that easily sabotage our efforts.

One individual who stands out for her devotion to the fight on obesity and inactivity is Cindy Boggs. Her long term commitment led me to appoint her to the Governor's Healthy Lifestyles Coalition. There she serves under the direction of the First Lady to affect policy and bring about positive change within school, business and community environments.

Cindy believes information is the missing link to achieving health goals. This was her motivation to create a Q and A fitness and health column, *CindySays*, which has been a popular resource since 2002 in the Charleston *Sunday Gazette-Mail.* Responding to countless inquiries about common challenges and misconceptions has given her great insight into the fitness industry with the ability to offer sound and reliable advice.

Now, she has written her first book, *CindySays – "You Can Find Health in Your Hectic World".* In this accessible book, she brings together her many years of YMCA experience as program developer, instructor trainer, fitness presenter, advice columnist and community health advocate to reach people where they live. She responds to the real questions and conflicts busy people face in their attempt to maintain a healthy lifestyle. Her insights not only reflect extensive knowledge and practical experience, but also understanding. She knows people, and it is this quality that sets Cindy apart.

We are fortunate that she has brought all of her experience and knowledge to bear on this easy-to-use, wide-ranging resource guide. We are proud that it has come from a native and lifelong West Virginian.

Therefore, it gives Gayle and me great pleasure to welcome her book, *CindySays – "You Can Find Health in Your Hectic World"*, as the healthy lifestyle advice book we all need.

In the interest of the best health for all of us,

**Joe Manchin III**

**Governor**

**Gayle C. Manchin**

**First Lady**

# Introduction

## "I'll Do Anything to Get Into Shape."
...overheard from so many desperate health-seekers

## "Okay-But Instead of Anything-Do the Right Thing."
...CindySays®

### Good News—Good Health

I've had the good fortune of working in the fitness industry for more than 25 years. I consider it a blessing because I've earned a living taking care of my mind, body and spirit. In addition, it has provided me insight into the obstacles many face in pursuit of an energetic life. I've observed enthusiastic exercisers without direction become exhausted in their efforts and fade away from the gym. I've witnessed men and women make New Year's resolutions only to drop them by mid-February. I've also watched committed people go at their workouts so hard they are forced to stop due to injury.

### Dazed and Confused

Early on, it was apparent to me that a well-meaning fitness industry could be a health seeker's biggest enemy. Staying up with the ever-changing trends, products and diets left most people dazed with confusion. Conflicting opinions, slick advertising campaigns and a hopeful public searching for the shortest path to health are at times, a recipe for disappointment. Too often, after repeated failure to reach goals, fitness and all that goes with it are put back on the shelf for another day.

## Let's Cut to the Chase

**As a writer in the fitness world,** I continually seek common sense answers to questions on health matters. My allegiance is to the needs of health-seekers rather than to fitness hype and merchandise. My advice is founded in science and tempered with an understanding that our lives are so hectic we must find simple strategies to better health. I find it a privilege to demystify the myriad of information fed to us each day, which is why I offer healthy lifestyle advice with a consumer-advocate mindset.

# Why Can't I Get Fit and Healthy?

- Do you wish you could wake up each day and feel confident you are living your healthiest life?
- Are you uncomfortable in the presence of fit people and the conversations they have?
- In your quest for a healthier life are you practicing more of a "hit and miss" strategy—with more misses than hits?

*Obviously you're interested—you ARE reading this*—so I want to make certain you are successful in your pursuit. This book will sort out confusing information that serve as roadblocks to your health and provide sensible answers to questions to facilitate a better life for you and your loved ones.

## I am So Frustrated!

*Few will argue that living healthfully in our hectic world is a challenge*—a challenge most never conquer. Lives are so frenzied; we are driven to find new ways of multi-tasking so we can squeeze more into our day. Families spend more time delegating responsibilities than they do enjoying their lives together.

*This same frantic existence has taken a huge toll on us nutritionally.* Drive-through dining has become the norm for many. New diets are born daily and even if we knew what was best for us--we have no time to shop, no time to prepare and often no time to sit down and enjoy a meal with our family.

*Add to this,* the countless amounts of health and fitness information thrown at us by companies and individuals, all with self-serving agendas. In our desperate search for health, we buy into one product and service after another. Too often we come away from each attempt a little more frustrated and a little less motivated.

## The Answers are Here

*I invite you to seek answers to your questions in this resource and help yourself to simple strategies toward realizing your health and fitness goals.* I am confident you can find health in your hectic world. It is completely accomplishable—in fact, it usually can be attained by altering just two or three things in your life. This may mean abandoning a bad habit and adopting a good one. But, it starts by valuing yourself and realizing that it is YOU—*not your husband, your wife, your mother, your boss, your friend*—who is in charge of devising a plan for a healthy life.

# IT'S NEVER 2 EARLY OR...2 LATE 4 BETTER HEALTH

## THE QUALITY OF YOUR LIFE DEPENDS ON IT

### FURTHERMORE...
### YOUR CHILDREN ARE WATCHING

Whether you're 18 or 80 now is the time to change the rest of your life. Information is the key to choosing and performing activity that is most advantageous to your body.

- ✓ Find the **BEST** health and fitness plan for your life.
- ✓ Set the **BEST** example to those you value and love.
- ✓ Be the **BEST** you can be starting today!

# Table of Contents

## Introduction
"I'll Do Anything to Get in Shape"

## Chapter One ............................................................................ 1-28
Health and Fitness Basics

## Chapter Two ......................................................................... 29-52
Great Arms, Firm Butts and Trim Waists

## Chapter Three ...................................................................... 53-84
The Right Type of Training for Me

## Chapter Four ....................................................................... 85-130
Injury, Illness and Limitation

## Chapter Five ...................................................................... 131-146
Fitness Gadgets and the Magic Bullet

## Chapter Six ........................................................................ 147-174
The Skinny on Eating for Health

## Chapter Seven ................................................................... 175-182
CindySays…"Final Thoughts"

## Glossary ............................................................................ 183-192
Get to Know Your Fitness and Health Terms

# Chapter Questions

## Chapter One
**Health and Fitness Basics**

- Q1. How Can Being Sedentary Harm Me?
- Q2. Am I Working Out Hard Enough for Results?
- Q3. How Much Exercise is Too Much?
- Q4. I Just Started Exercising—Why Does it Hurt So Much?
- Q5. Is it Important to Know How Much Body Fat I Have?
- Q6. What's the Most Accurate Way to Measure Body Fat?
- Q7. What's the Importance of a Resting Heart Rate?
- Q8. I've Never Stretched—So Why Now?
- Q9. Why Can't I Stick to an Exercise Plan?
- Q10. Should Older Adults Weight Train?
- Q11. What Is the Most Valuable Element for Good Health?
- Q12. How Can I Help my Overweight Child?
- Q13. How Much Physical Activity Do I Have to Do?

# Chapter Two
## Great Arms, Firm Butts and Trim Waists

- (14) How Can I Trim my Waist?
- (15) How Can I Firm Up my Butt?
- (16) Cardio and Strength—What's the Perfect Mix?
- (17) How Do I Strengthen My Abs on a Big Ball?
- (18) How Can I Reduce the Fat Around my Hips?
- (19) What Are the Best Exercises for Great Arms?
- (20) How Can I Lose Weight?
- (21) How Do I Get Back in Shape after Pregnancy?
- (22) How Do I Get Muscle Definition?

# Chapter Three
## The Right Type of Training for Me

- (23) Do I Need a Personal Trainer?
- (24) How Do I Become a Better Runner?
- (25) How Do I Train to Become a Better Skier?
- (26) Are Pilates and Yoga Alike?
- (27) What Can Pilates Do for Me?
- (28) How Do I Know if I Have a Bad Personal Trainer?

29 Am I a Bad Personal Training Client?

30 What is Isometric Exercise?

31 How Can I Do Step Aerobics Safely?

32 What is Functional Training?

33 How Do I Get Better at Racquet Sports?

34 How Do I Train for Speed and Quickness?

35 How Do I Train to Be a Better Cyclist?

36 Can I Add Too Much Muscle to my Body?

37 How Can I Improve my Balance?

# Chapter Four
## Injury, Illness and Limitation

38 What Causes Shin Splints?

39 How Do I Prevent Backaches?

40 What Exercise is Helpful for Scoliosis?

41 I Have Plantar Fasciitis—What Can I Do?

42 My Knees Hurt—How Can I Stay Active?

43 I Have Osteoporosis—Can Exercise Help?

44 Can Swimming Help Rebuild my Bones?

45 How Can I Stay Active with Osteoarthritis?

Q46 How Can I Exercise with Urinary Incontinence?

Q47 What Can I Do about Tennis Elbow?

Q48 Will Resistance Training Help Diabetics?

Q49 How Do I Exercise with Rheumatoid Arthritis?

Q50 Why Do My Bendable Parts Crack and Pop?

Q51 Can I Resume Exercise after Cancer Treatment?

Q52 How Can I Ease the Pain in my Side when I Run?

Q53 How Do I Exercise Safely in the Heat?

Q54 What Are Good Exercises for People with MS?

Q55 I Have Varicose Veins—Should I Exercise?

Q56 How Do I Avoid the Germs in the Gym?

Q57 Should I Work Out When I am Sick?

# Chapter Five

## Fitness Gadgets and the Magic Bullet

Q58 Do Ab Exercisers Really Work?

Q59 Who or What is a Bosu Trainer?

Q60 Why Buy Resistance Bands if I Have Weights?

Q61 What Is a Rebounder?

Q62 Should I Join the Dance Dance Revolution?

(63) Are Cardiovascular Machines Worth Buying?

(64) How Can a Heart Rate Monitor Help Me?

(65) What Is a Power Plate and Does It Work?

(66) What Home Equipment Should I Invest in?

# Chapter Six

## The Skinny on Eating for Health

(67) How Can the New Food Pyramid Help me?

(68) What is the Bottom Line on Low-Carb Diets?

(69) How Do I Snack Healthfully?

(70) How Much Protein Do I Need Each Day?

(71) I Exercise Regularly—Am I Entitled to Dessert?

(72) How Do I Stop Overeating at Holiday Time?

(73) I Love Buffets—How Can I Avoid Them?

(74) How Do I Avoid Gaining Weight in College?

(75) What Should I Eat after a Workout?

(76) How Do I Keep my Child from Snacking?

(77) What's the Quickest Diet Fix?

(78) What Does Low-Glycemic and High-Glycemic Mean?

# Chapter Seven
## CindySays...Final Thoughts

- How Do I Stick with my Healthy Lifestyle?
- Valuable Insight from my Mentors

# Chapter 1

# HEALTH AND FITNESS BASICS

**Gee, if only I had known that!** Little things mean a lot. Enough small changes can add up to large improvements with regard to looking good and feeling great. Stumbling blocks in the form of confusion, intimidation, misinformation, or the abundance of bad advice can make you throw in the towel. Most of the time, just having clear-cut information and confidence can make the difference between making exercise work in your life and eliminating it from life's to-do list.

**You've made the first step.** You've purchased your fitness center membership, picked up the newest shoes and athletic wear on the market…uh hum….now what? What do I do?—where do I start? It can be a daunting task to sort out the myriad of choices on a fitness center's menu. There should always be knowledgeable staff on hand to help you… but what if you don't know exactly what to ask?

**A good start begins with good information.** This chapter will fill you in on the basics of health and fitness. It will supply you with the facts you need to work smart…to work efficiently and to avoid common pitfalls that undermine and delay healthy results.

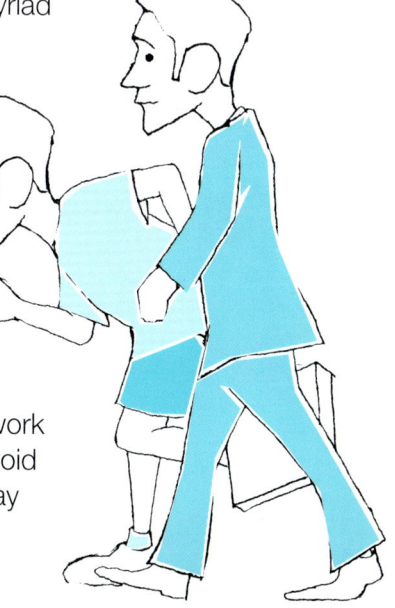

# Q1 How Can Being Sedentary Harm Me?

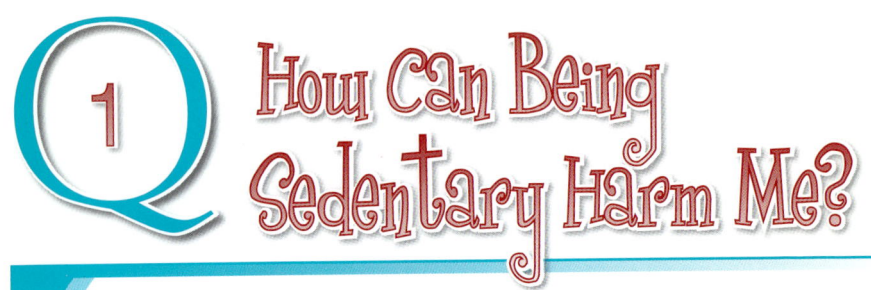

**A sedentary lifestyle**—one that does not include regular exercise either at work or at home—will ultimately cause your cardiovascular and respiratory systems (heart and lungs) to become progressively weaker each day.

- Muscles will atrophy (shrink away)
- Joints will stiffen and lose their range of motion
- Your entire body will be easily injured
- Your risk of heart disease, high blood pressure, cancer, diabetes, osteoporosis, fatigue and obesity will increase

## Just 30 Minutes of Moderate Exercise Most Days of the Week Will

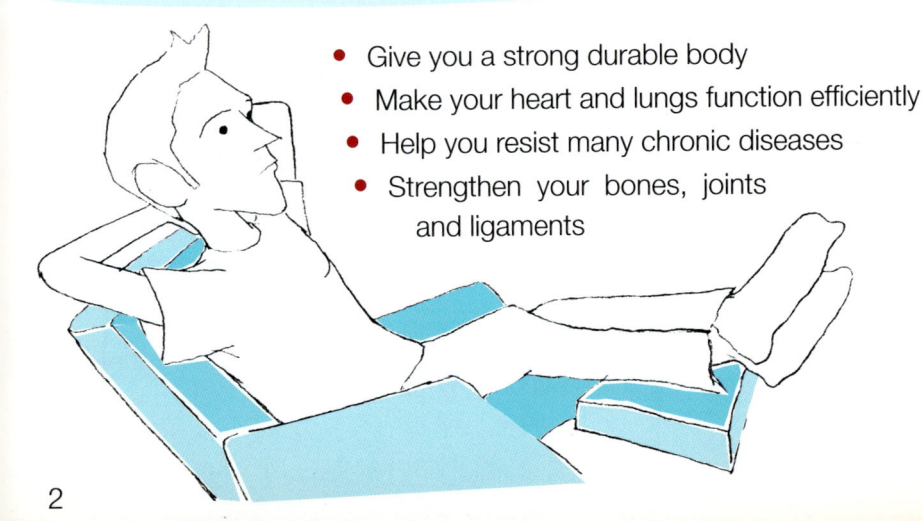

- Give you a strong durable body
- Make your heart and lungs function efficiently
- Help you resist many chronic diseases
- Strengthen your bones, joints and ligaments

- Enable you to manage your weight
- Preserve good posture
- Make you sleep better
- Perk up your immune system
- Build self-esteem and confidence
- Resist the aging process

Take a walk, ride a bike, swim, do anything that gets you moving. Your quality and quantity of life depends on it.

# Q2 Am I Working Out Hard Enough for Results?

In order for your physical activity to give you great results, it must be difficult enough to challenge your heart and lungs but not so difficult it creates a safety risk. There are several ways to verify activity effectiveness by **monitoring your intensity**.

1. The easiest and least accurate is the *"Talk Test"* method. If you are able to sing while exercising, you are probably not working hard enough. If you have an *increase in breathing rate but are able to talk, you are probably in an ideal range.* If you are gasping for air and unable to talk, you are working too hard for aerobic benefits.

2. The Borg Scale uses a *(RPE) Rating of Perceived Exertion* to monitor intensity. Using a self-rated scale from 6 to 20—6 being very, very light intensity and 20 being maximum intensity—each number is associated with how you feel. *Ratings between 12 to14* on the Borg Scale indicate a moderate level of physical activity.

3. The *(THR) Target Heart Rate* method predicts how hard a person should be working based on age and suggests an appropriate heart rate range. Your *(MHR) Maximum Heart Rate* must be determined by subtracting your age from 220. Finding 60% and 80% of this number will give you a *(THRR) Target Heart Rate Range*, which is generally a safe and effective intensity.

4. The *Karvonen* method is more accurate because it factors in not only the exerciser's age, but also, their fitness level, using their

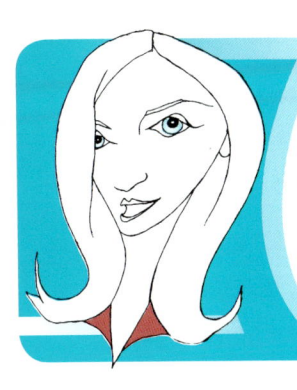

**CindySays...** *"For an effortless way to accurately check your pulse during activity, you may want to consider wearing a heart rate monitor. They consist of a small strap worn under your exercise clothes and a handy wrist band with an easy to read display."*

*(RHR) Resting Heart Rate.* Do this by taking your pulse (heart rate) for a full minute upon waking and while completely still. Repeat and record this for a week and then average the numbers. This will determine your RHR.

## LET'S SEE HOW THIS WORKS WITH BOTH FORMULAS

### Target Heart Rate Formula- (Basic)

220 – AGE = ____ X 60% = YOUR LOW RANGE

220 – AGE = ____ X 80% = YOUR HIGH RANGE

### Example for 40-Year-Old- Factoring in ONLY age

220 – 40 = 180  X  60% = 108 YOUR LOW RANGE

220 – 40 = 180  X  80% = 144 YOUR HIGH RANGE

**This 40-year-old would have a THRR of 108 to 144**

## Karvonen Formula (Influenced by Fitness Level)

220 – AGE = ___ - RHR = ___ X 60% = ___ + RHR = YOUR LOW RANGE
220 – AGE = ___ - RHR = ___ X 80% = ___ + RHR = YOUR HIGH RANGE

## The Same 40-Year-Old Factoring in a RHR of 65

220 – 40 = 180 – 65 = 115 X 60% = 69 + 65 = 134 YOUR LOW RANGE
220 – 40 = 180 – 65 = 115 X 80% = 92 + 65 = 157 YOUR HIGH RANGE

**This 40-year-old would have a THRR of 134 to 157**

In both formulas, these Two Numbers will set your parameters for challenging yet safe exercise. However, you can see by using the Karvonen method and factoring in a resting heart rate (fitness level) the THRR changes. It is personalized and will suggest a more accurate range. Memorize these numbers, so you can monitor the effectiveness of your intensity at any time by taking your pulse for 6 seconds and multiplying it by 10.

## THINGS YOU SHOULD KNOW ABOUT HEART RATES

**❶** For greater accuracy start counting your pulse with zero instead of one

**❷** Taking your pulse is a good place to start, but is only accurate to within plus or minus 12 beats per minute

**❸** Many prescription and non-prescription medications can alter your heart rhythm or rate

# Q3 How Much Exercise Is Too Much?

**As with everything in life**, too much of any "good" thing can be a "bad" thing. Exercise is an essential ingredient of a healthy life for both physical and mental fitness. However, if you're feeling guilty over missing a workout or use your activity as penance for overeating, you may be missing all the wonderful benefits exercise can offer.

## If You Are Not Over-Exercising

- Exercising will leave you invigorated, strong, and feeling rejuvenated
- Mild muscle soreness should be brief and should be easily traced back to a specific exercise that you performed.
- You will feel a positive effect on both mind and spirit if exercise is thought of as a supplement to your life and not your entire life.

## If You Are Over-Exercising

- Workouts are making you weak and/or fatigued
- Not working out may leave you guilt-ridden
- Failure to reach fitness goals makes you irritated
- You may be experiencing constant pain or discomfort in your joints
- You may be neglecting other important obligations with family and work

These are signs that a person is working out to excess. If so, it will be necessary to ask yourself why you are exercising in order to make changes that will lead to more balance in your training and ultimately your life.

# Q4 I Just Started Exercising- Why Does it Hurt So Much?

**Ouch!** This painful consequence is commonly known as **DOMS—Delayed Onset Muscle Soreness**. It happens when you introduce your body to physical activity that is new or different—perhaps a new sport, a new class, a new mountain, or a new intensity of something familiar.

This type of muscle pain is sneaky—most people are pain free during the initial activity as the pain lies in wait for 12 to 24 hours. Then it hits and hangs around for as long as three or four days. It can make you feel like you've been run over by a truck—complete with aching, stiffness, and a total lack of desire to move.

### There Are Ways To Ease and/or Shorten DOMS:

- Warm up for 5 to 10 minutes before activity
- Cool down for 5 to 10 minutes following activity
- Spend at least 5 minutes stretching after exercise
- Start new activity gradually and slowly add time and intensity
- Strength training should start with minimal amounts of resistance focusing on form and posture
- Gradually progress the amount of weight you lift to allow muscle adaptation

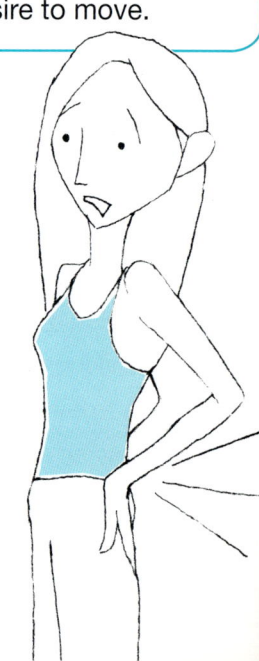

## *Belated Advice If You Are Already In Pain:*

- Rest and apply ice to sore areas
- Gentle stretches and massage promote healing
- Non-steroidal anti-inflammatory medication like aspirin or ibuprofen may alleviate pain
- Do some easy low-impact exercise to increase blood flow to the affected muscles
- Some evidence shows vitamin C to decrease soreness
- If pain persists past seven days consult a physician or physical therapist

Be assured, this response to unusual exertion is quite normal and will subside. The muscles will adapt to the new stress. In fact, this adaptation is precisely what leads to increased muscle strength and endurance.

# Q5: Is it Important to Know How Much Body Fat I Have?

It is if you are interested in your health. Body weight tells you what your skin and everything inside it weighs. Your body is made of two types of material. One type is lean muscle, which is **metabolically active**, and the other is body fat, which is **metabolically inactive**—added together make up your body weight. Body composition essentially measures each of these separately and tells you how much lean muscle compared to body fat you have.

*Metabolically Active* - Muscle, bone, organs, ligaments, and tendons comprise the largest part of this type of tissue. They require calories to stay in good working order. The more muscle you have, the more calories your body burns.

*Metabolically Inactive* - Adipose or fat comprise this type of tissue. Your body requires a minimal amount (essential fats) for health but too much is associated with illness and disease. The more fat you have, the fewer calories your body burns.

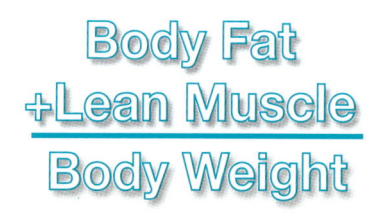

Body Fat
+Lean Muscle
Body Weight

## How Much Body Fat Should I Have?

| Classification | Women (% Fat) | Men (% Fat) |
| --- | --- | --- |
| Essential Fat | 10-12 percent | 2-4 percent |
| Athletes | 14-20 percent | 6-13 percent |
| Fitness | 21-24 percent | 14-17 percent |
| Acceptable | 25-31 percent | 18-25 percent |

You should know that over 25% body fat for men and over 32% body fat for women increases the risk for weight-related illness such as high blood pressure, heart disease, diabetes, gallstones, osteoarthritis and some cancers.

# Q6 What's the Most Accurate Way to Measure Body Fat?

## Most Accurate

**1** ***DEXA*** (dual energy X-ray absorptiometry) scan is the gold standard for determining body fat. This is an x-ray machine specifically for bone density but can also measure body fat. Though usually expensive, it can provide you with a precise body fat result with a 1 to 3 percent margin of error.

**2** ***Hydrostatic*** or underwater weighing is another accurate way to calculate body fat. This method is also costly and not readily available. Since you must exhale all the air from your lungs as you are immersed in a hydrostatic weighing tank, it can also be intimidating and exhaustive.

## Most Practical

**1** ***Skinfold Measurement*** is slightly less accurate but more practical. A special caliper (pincher-like device) pinches your skin in specific locations on your body and measures the amount of fat you have under your skin. Most gyms or health clubs use this cost-effective method which is reliable when done correctly by experienced professionals.

**2** ***Bioelectrical Impedance*** is one of the quickest methods of measuring body fat. Handheld and standing scale models measure the speed at which a low-level electrical signal passes through your body. It can be reasonably accurate but can be adversely affected by various factors such as recent physical activity, skin temperature and hydration levels during the test.

## Is Accuracy Everything?

*No*—keeping track of body fat is a great way to stay in touch with your overall health profile because this measurement tells you how much fat and muscle comprise your body. However, body fat tests do not need to be 100% accurate. They simply need to be regular so you may use this calculation as an ongoing reference to monitor your exercise progression. Body composition does not change quickly, so checking it every eight to ten weeks is sufficient.

# Q7 What's the Importance of a Resting Heart Rate?

**The Resting Heart Rate (RHR)**—a person's heart rate at rest—represents the minimum number of heart beats needed to sustain the body. Perceiving your body's intensity throughout any activity is key to working in a safe and proper range. Working at an optimum intensity will give you the kind of results you want without jeopardizing your health.

Your RHR is a fairly accurate indicator of your fitness level. The lower your resting heart rate is, the stronger your heart is—conversely, the faster it is, the less efficient it is at circulating blood to and from your heart. It is a good idea to know your resting heart rate. The best time to find out your resting heart rate is in the morning, after a good night's sleep, and before you get out of bed.

## Resting Heart Rate Facts

- An average heart beats about 60 to 80 times a minute while at rest
- Resting heart rates usually rise with age
- Resting heart rates over 70 have a greater risk of heart attack than those below 70
- Cardiovascular training lowers your resting heart rate

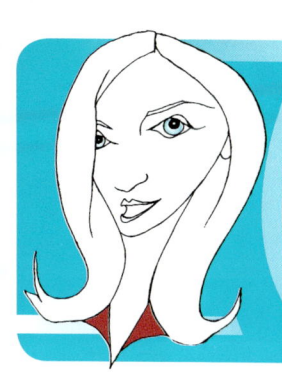

**CindySays**..."*Place a watch with a second hand beside your bed at night so when you wake to take your RHR you won't have to rise—you can remain still for a more accurate heart rate reading.*"

## Here's How to Determine Your Resting Heart Rate

**❶** Take your pulse just after waking in the morning while you are lying still

**❷** Count the beats for a full minute

**❸** Repeat this five consecutive days

**❹** Add the five resting heart rates together and divide by five to obtain your resting heart rate

**❺** Always take your resting heart rate under the same conditions to ensure accuracy

# Q8 I've Never Stretched- So Why Now?

**Some people seem to defy the odds** and get by with minimal or hit and miss stretching. Eventually though, luck runs out and you will be at greater risk for injury. You must stretch if you want to maintain flexibility and enjoy an active life.

**Too many people make the mistake** of stretching prior to exercise. This is ineffective at best and can possibly be injurious. Connective tissue surrounds your muscles and is not supple when cold. The best time to stretch is when your body is warm.

## Most Common Types of Stretches

- *Dynamic Stretching*-muscles are engaged in gentle movement for a progressive increase in range of motion. Example- WALKING LUNGE

- *Static Stretching*- a stretch taken to a point of resistance, but without pain or movement. Maintain mild tension for 10 to 30 seconds, rest and repeat. Example- RELAXED TOE TOUCHES

- *Active Stretching*- muscles are placed in a position of tension and held without assistance. Example- YOGA POSES

- *Passive Stretching*- a relaxed stretch in which you are assisted by your own body weight or an external force to reach a full range of motion. Example-ASSISTED PARTNER STRETCHES

- *Ballistic Stretching*- uses the momentum of a moving body or a limb in an attempt to force it beyond its normal range of motion. Stretching by bouncing into (or out of) a stretched position, using the stretched muscles as a spring which pulls you out of the stretched position can lead to injury. It does not allow your muscles to relax in the stretched position. It may instead cause them to tighten by repeatedly activating the stretch reflex. Example-REPEATEDLY BOUNCING DOWN TO TOUCH YOUR TOES

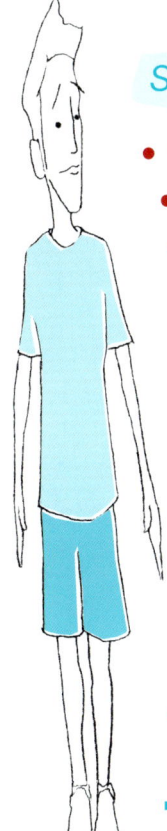

## Stretching Tips

- Warm body up with brisk walk or light jog prior to stretch
- Stretch after each workout
- Stretches should be performed with gradual progression without bouncing
- Move to a point of mild tension and hold for 15 to 60 seconds
- There should never be pain associated with a stretch
- Diligent stretching decreases likelihood of muscle injury and imbalances
- Accompanying each stretch with relaxation breathing will yeild better results
- Avoid stretching injured muscles or joints unless directed by physician
- Stretch to reduce post-workout muscle fatigue and soreness

# Q9 Why can't I stick to an Exercise Plan?

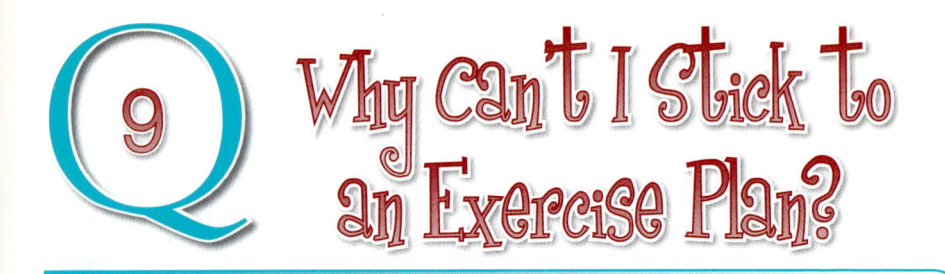

**Making exercise a natural part of your lifestyle** is about decision making. The activities you fill your time with will usually be ones you look forward to and enjoy. Working out is no different. Some start an activity because their friends are doing it, the gym is convenient, or is held at an opportune time. If the kind of exercise you choose isn't based on YOU, it probably won't stick. This is merely the failure to match your energy level and personality to the right type of activity.

## Ask Yourself These Questions

- Are you self-motivated?
- Are you shy or are you social?
- Do you thrive on or avoid competition?
- Are you cautious or adventurous?
- How much time are you willing to devote to activity?
- What activities naturally attract you?

If you are a nature lover or an adventurer, you are probably not going to love being in a gym setting all the time. Try hiking, cycling, mountain biking, canoeing, rock climbing, skiing, or Tai chi. On the other hand, if you enjoy being around people, the gym may be just the place to workout.

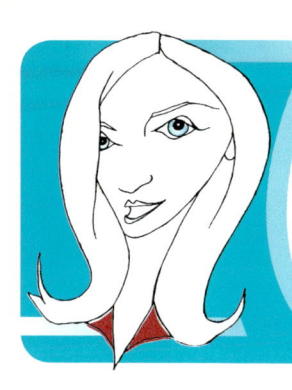

**CindySays**..."*Begin viewing exercise as you would a doctor's appointment, a conference with your child's teacher, or key business meeting—make it a valuable priority.*"

If you are self-motivated and love to challenge your limits, weight training, jogging, tennis, golf, martial arts, or yoga may be your ticket to consistency. Perhaps you are social and enjoy being part of a team. Look for group-oriented activities such as sports, water aerobics, fitness classes, walking or dance clubs.

### Different activity may attract you at different times of your life.

Look for your interests to change periodically based on time constraints, family duties, abilities, desires, and energy levels. For example, you may want to take up golf but recognize your inability to devote four to six hours from your day due to family and/or work obligations. Tennis, which will give you comparable challenges in an hour or two, may be a better choice at this time of your life.

### Exercise must be enjoyable

Chances are if you're not having fun, you won't keep scheduling activity into your hectic lifestyle. Choose activities that are compatible with your personality. Idle choices will get you nowhere—thoughtful choices will keep you moving in the right direction.

# Q10 Should Older Adults Weight Train?

**Some people believe** lifting when you are an older adult may damage joints and ligaments. However, if no joint problems are present; lifting weights as we age is the secret to healthy bones, joints and ligaments and brings about many positive benefits.

This is not to say that someone who has never been involved with weight training or resistance work should just buy a set of weights or jump on a machine and get going. That kind of hap hazard approach to strength training *could result* in damage to tendons and ligaments at any age.

## Safe Steps for Safe Weight Training

- Visit your health care professional for a physical exam and permission to begin
- Identify limitations such as joint pain, arthritis, or past injuries
- Record any recommendations or restrictions
- Consult a certified fitness professional such as a physical therapist or personal trainer for thorough evaluation to establish fitness goals and review limitations
- Come away with a personalized strength training program so you may work smart and avoid unnecessary stress to the joints

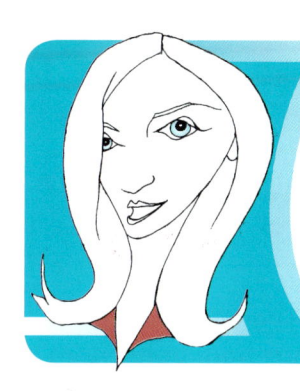

***CindySays***... *"In addition to building a healthier body, you will also be preventing osteoporosis (loss of bone density) — one of the most debilitating diseases facing older adults."*

## *This Program Would Outline In Writing*

- Appropriate pre-workout exercises to prepare your body
- Each exercise necessary for each muscle group
- Amount of weight for each exercise
- Total repetitions for each exercise (*number of times you lift a weight*)
- Total number of sets for each exercise (*number of times you repeat the repetitions*)
- Correct exercise form and posture
- Proper breathing technique
- Lifting speed and range of motion
- Number of workouts per week necessary for functional benefits
- Modifications regarding any existing limitations
- Post-workout stretching and range of motion exercises

Once familiar with your detailed program you will be well equipped to continue on your own in a supervised atmosphere. Your joints and ligaments will become healthier and stronger in response to strength training if you perform the exercises safely within a properly prescribed program.

# Q11 What is the Most Valuable Element for Good Health?

There is not just one but rather three. There should be a disciplined approach with regard to **good nutrition, consistent physical activity, and stress management**. One without the others throws the balance of health off. Each of these components is dependent on the others.

Discipline is the key word here, which establishes a sense of control, restraint, order, or consistency. Without discipline, the opposite will describe your life—chaos, bedlam, disorder, or turmoil.

## A DISCIPLINED APPROACH

### Nutrition

- Pay attention to portion control and a balance of calories
- Eat 5 to 6 small meals a day
- Eat nutrient dense foods
- Eat good carbohydrates such as fresh fruits, vegetables and whole grains
- Choose lean protein and eat small amounts with each meal
- Drink lots of water

## Physical Activity

- Move your body 30 to 40 minutes most days of the week
- Alternate days of cardiovascular exercise and strength training
- Warm up 5 to 10 minutes before your workout
- Cool down 5 to 10 minutes after your workout
- Stretch muscles thoroughly after any physical activity
- Avoid boredom by varying your workouts every 6 to 8 weeks

## Stress Management

- Set aside quiet time for yourself each day even if for only 10 minutes
- Practice emptying your mind of obligation
- Deep breath periodically throughout each day and as you fall asleep
- Learn a practice like yoga, Pilates, Tai Chi or meditation
- Create a pleasant home and work environment
- Treat yourself to a long bath or massage to relax and restore your mind and body

# Q12 How Can I Help my Overweight Child?

**It's a catch-22** that goes something like this. A child who is slightly overweight soon opts for less and less activity until no longer comfortable with activity. They find themselves trapped in a sedentary lifestyle, unable and unmotivated to find a way out.

Pointing them in the direction of competitive sports is like expecting them to be excited about jumping from an airplane without a parachute. They are not equipped and they know it. Being fairly adept at predicting their future they understandably turn away from anything they see themselves failing at. Children who view themselves as overweight and non-competitive often usually struggle with self-confidence issues.

## There Are Some Doable Solutions

- Non-competitive activities that can be learned alone such as *bowling, hiking, kayaking, tennis or one of the many types of self-defense*
- Family exercise such as *walking or riding a bike*
- For children eight and older — *supervised strength training*

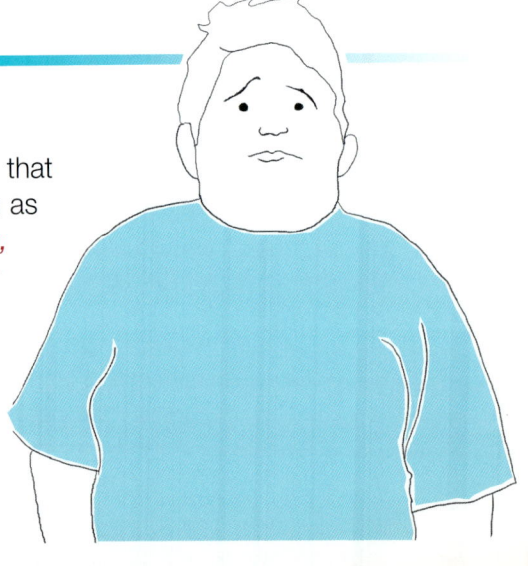

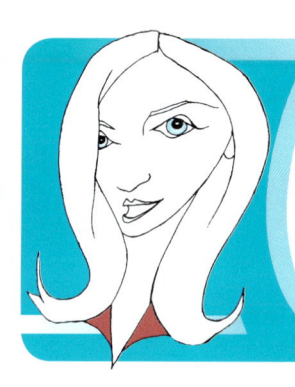

***CindySays***... *"Children participating in a sensible and supervised strength training program develop positive attitudes toward exercise therefore stand a better chance of adopting healthier lifestyles."*

## Strength Training Can Be a Great Solution Because it Builds

- Strong muscles
- Strong bones
- Self-esteem

**The goal in weight training children** is not muscle mass or as a means to a competitive end but rather for muscular endurance, co-ordination, weight control and improved confidence. Always talk with your medical professional before starting a new physical program with children who are overweight. If your child participates in a strength training program, make certain it is supervised at all times by a fitness professional. National guidelines for youth strength training have been established and should be followed.

# 13. How Much Physical Activity Do I Have to Do?

**Adults should plan to get at least 30 minutes** and children 60 minutes of moderate physical activity most days of the week to improve your health and to build resistance to disease. You may need more minutes for the prevention of weight gain, for weight loss, or to manage your weight.

One of the most common reasons people choose not to exercise is that they believe they lack the time and/or energy to get a workout in. **Physical activity is CUMULATIVE!** In other words, if you have 10 minutes in the morning, 15 minutes on your lunch hour, and 20 minutes in the evening, you can claim a workout.

## Consider Using Your Time and Energy Wisely

### Morning (10 Minute Options)

- Climb your stairs two at a time
- Take a brisk walk
- Slip in a short yoga workout

### Afternoon (15 Minute Options)

- Walk with a co-worker
- Keep weights at work for squats, lunges, shoulder presses, biceps and triceps
- Do as many push-ups as you can and follow with a thorough stretch

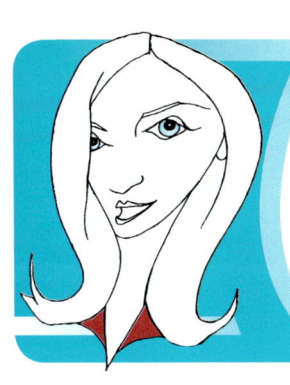

***CindySays***..."Look for opportunities for physical activity. Your minutes can be cumulative. Moving your body for 10, 15 or 20 minutes can be the difference between a sedentary life and an active one. Change the pace of your life."

## *Evening (20 Minute Options)*

- Ride a bike
- Jog or walk briskly
- Participate in an activity with your children or grandchildren
- Use an exercise ball for core work and stretching
- Dance with lively music
- Climb your stairs and lift weights or use resistance band
- Practice Pilates or yoga

## Chapter 2

# GREAT ARMS-FIRM BUTTS-TRIM WAISTS

**What do you mean I can't spot reduce?** I mean you can't spot reduce. If people could spot reduce, then you would see professional tennis players swinging their racquet from a tiny REDUCED arm. A tennis player's dominant arm gets about as much training as any targeted butt or hips ever could have. It will definitely get stronger and increase lean tissue…however; the overlying fat disappears only when the body is in calorie deficit.

**In other words**, a body must be expending more calories than it is ingesting in order to lose excess fat. Even then, it will lose it throughout the entire body—and is unrelated to specific problem areas that are being trained.

**So how do we improve our butts**, guts and other assorted body parts? We strengthen these areas by targeting movement and resistance to muscle. These areas adapt and respond by building healthy muscle tissue along with better joint integrity.

**Working toward better muscular strength and endurance** will produce durable bodies. Add to that a nutrient rich diet and those once troublesome areas begin to shed excess fat. Because fallacy and fitness team up so often together, chapter two offers insight into truth, training and the pursuit of great parts.

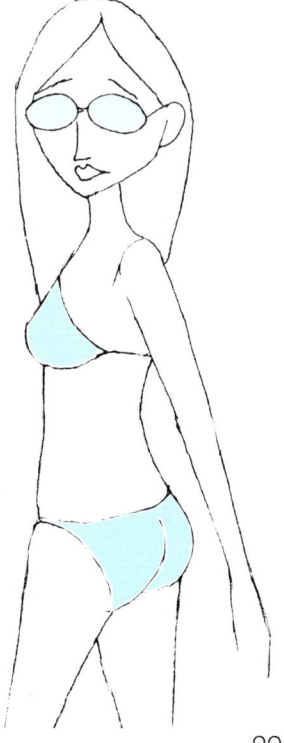

# Q14 How Can I Trim My Waist?

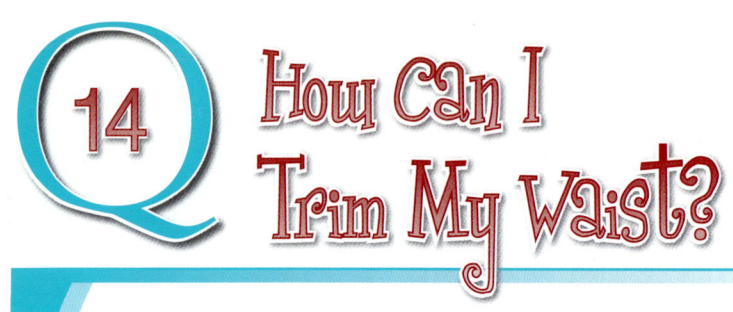

**A thick mid-section** is usually caused by excess fat around the middle and is somewhat predetermined based on hereditary factors. Little can be done when it comes to changing inherited traits. However, cardiovascular work to burn calories and (high repetition/low weight) strength training to increase metabolism and produce long lean muscles is your best bet for a slimmer waist.

## Diet and Exercise

- Cardiovascular training most days of the week
- Strength training upper and lower body
- Limit saturated fats and empty calories (sweets and sodas)
- Do consume lean meat, fish, whole grains, fresh fruits, vegetables and water

## Workout

- Strengthen overall musculature concentrating on medial deltoids to broaden shoulders and create illusion of smaller waist
- Weight-free abdominal crunches on a large balance ball-curling straight up

- Oblique crunches-curling up with a slight trunk rotation alternating each side
- Pilates Class would be class of choice when your goal is to train the core

## *Big Mistake*

- A poor choice of exercise to trim the waist is a side bend with high weight. Not only is this potentially dangerous for your back, this type of training may increase the size of your waist.

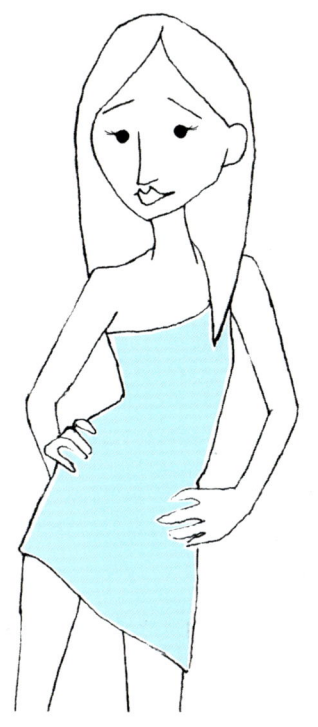

# Q15 How Can I Firm Up My Butt?

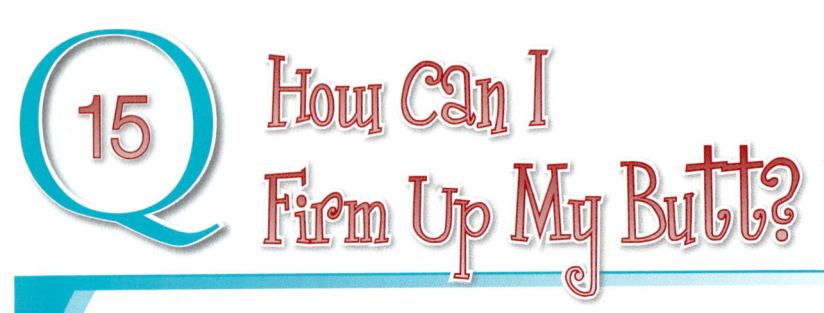

**Regarding the butt**, women are quick to use descriptions such as—dropped, sagging, too flat, too wide, and too soft. "Butt" make no mistake about it...the key word is "Up". Apparently, the way we fill out our jeans—or don't—ranks high on the self-esteem priority list.

## Here Are the Best Butt Exercises

- *Cardio—Moderate to Steep Incline Walking and Sprinting*—this will burn calories and tighten those muscles. Blend this into your cardiovascular workouts 3 times a week. Check out the backside of sprinters if you want to see well-defined glutes. The incline or hill will encourage extra muscle recruitment of the glutes.

- *Strength Work— Prone Leg Lifts Over a Ball*—Lie with stomach down on a large exercise ball and place hands on the floor. After tightening your gluteals, lift one leg slightly off the floor, keeping leg straight. Then alternate sides. *As this exercise becomes easier, try lifting both legs simultaneously*—but only if you can do it without feeling strain in your back.

- *Strength Work—Lunge*—hold two dumbbells in your hands by your sides. Step forward with one leg (so your heel stays beneath your knee) and lower your upper body down until your bottom knee almost touches the ground. Do not allow your knee to go forward of your toes as you come down. Push up and back to starting position alternating

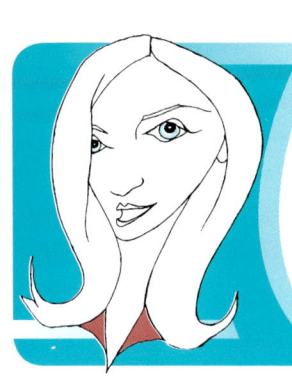

> **CindySays**..."The foods you eat will play an important role in determining results."

legs. The farther forward you step, the more the glutes and hamstrings you will use. *Keep your upper body vertical and spine straight.*

- *Strength Work—Full Squats*—stand with feet hip-width apart and squat, keeping back straight, abs in and knees behind your toes. Contract gluteals as you stand back up. With healthy knees, back and adequate flexibility this exercise will do wonders for your entire lower body. *Perfecting the full squat is a must for a great butt.*

- *Strength Work—Dead lifts*—stand with feet hip-width apart, weight in front of thighs. Keeping back flat and abdominals in, hinge forward from the hips and lower your torso until bar reaches mid-shin. Squeeze butt to bring yourself back to standing position. Keep the bar close to your legs through the entire movement and do not bend your knees. *The glutes require heavy loads for adequate stimulation but perfect execution is essential. *Nothing lifts the butt like a dead lift. *Keep legs straight only if you have a strong back and flexible hamstrings—if not, bend your knees slightly.*

- *Strength Work—Bridge*—Lie on your back with knees bent, feet on the floor and hip-width apart. Slowly peel your spine from the floor from the bottom one vertebra at a time, tightening the glutes and hamstrings until you've created a diagonal line from your shoulders to your knees. Return to the starting position slowly, one vertebra at a time. *This movement is great for your back also.*

The prototype for the perfect bottom is thankfully in the eye of the beholder. Some prefer slim hipped while others like curvaceous and round; some want an athletically toned tush while others are happy with plenty of junk in their trunk. No matter what your preference, your jeans are going to look their very best on a derriere that is continually "firmed up" by activity geared for the rear.

## Additional Activities to Build a Better Butt

- Swimming
- Biking
- Stepping
- Pilates
- Kickboxing

# Q16 Cardio and Strength What's the Perfect Mix?

**Both cardiovascular and strength training** are essential in a balanced workout plan. Too often weight training is overlooked as many devote a majority of their time to aerobic exercise. The perfect workout mix however, is a blend of cardio, strength and flexibility.

## For The Average Adult Pursuing General Fitness Conditioning

- 20-60 minutes of aerobic activity 3-5 days a week
- 20-30 minutes of weight training 2-3 times a week
- Deliberate stretches to increase range of motion following all physical activity

This is a great place to start. Now examine your particular goals so to fine tune a workout into the perfect mix for you. Ask yourself—is there a sport you are involved in or hoping to be? Do you have a deadline—for example a race you are preparing for? If so, then these are the criteria that will help determine how much aerobic activity you will do in comparison to weight training.

**In addition, clarify your priorities.** Consider how each of the following concerns is affected most by focusing on aerobic training or strength training. Keep in mind aerobic exercises are designed primarily to improve one muscle—your heart, strength training works on almost every muscle but the heart.

## *Focus by First Determining Your Needs*

- Bone Density—**DO MORE**—Strength Training
- Blood Pressure—**DO MORE**—Aerobics
- Resting Heart Rate—**DO MORE**—Aerobics
- Strength—**DO MORE**—Strength Training
- HDL Cholesterol—**DO MORE**—Aerobics
- Resting Metabolic Rate—**DO MORE**—Strength Training
- Appearance—**DO MORE**—Strength Training
- Body Composition—**DO MORE**—Strength Training
- Longevity—**DO MORE**—Aerobics

It is important to note that those who have established a clear purpose for their exercise are more likely to have more meaningful, effective workouts and better results

## Q17: How Do I Strengthen my Abs on a Big Ball?

**These big balls have many aliases**—*BALANCE BALL, SWISS BALL, EXERCISE BALL, GYM BALL, PILATES BALL, SPORTS BALL, FITNESS BALL, STABILITY BALL, THERAPY BALL, YOGA BALL, BODY BALL*—and deserve high marks for their ability to transform ordinary abdominal work into interesting and highly effective exercise. They offer cushioned support while they demand the user to engage the stabilizer muscles of the core. They intensify the work by recruiting more muscle fibers and improve muscle memory. This tends to give you faster and better results. The ball is also an excellent tool for stretching and a refreshing departure from so much equipment that promises everything and delivers nothing.

Healthy backs and abdominals (abs) allow your body to move with strength, balance, and grace. Two excellent exercise choices on the ball to strengthen these areas are the crunch and the back extension.

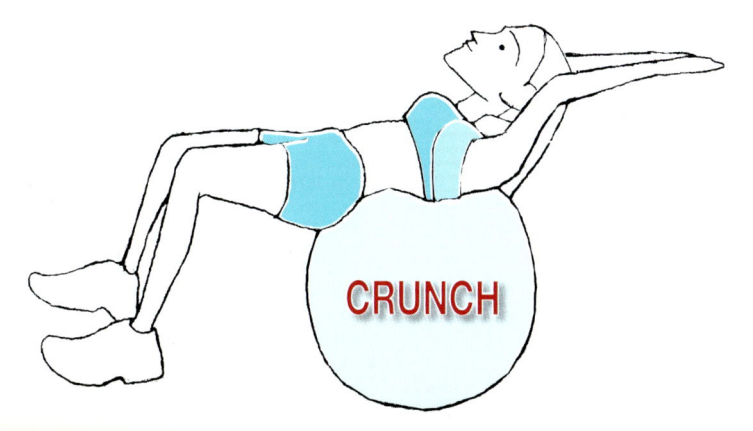

CRUNCH

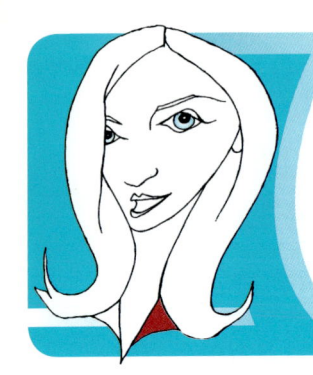

***CindySays***..."*One caveat—don't buy into the idea that all exercise should be done on a ball. It has specific uses and limitations. Appreciate what it does best—Abs and Backs!*"

SIZE MATTERS!!! Oftentimes people use poor form or an incorrect ball size which can lessen the effectiveness of the abdominal work and lead to back problems.

## *Choosing the Right Size Ball For You*

### *If Your Height is:*

- Less than 5' 0" Choose a 45cm ball
- 5' 0" to 5' 5" Choose a 55cm ball
- 5' 6" to 6' 1" Choose a 65cm ball
- 6' 2" to 6' 8" Choose a 75cm ball

### *Once Inflated Make Sure When Seated:*

- Knees and hips are at 90 degrees with thighs parallel to floor
- If hips are higher than knee level—ball is too large or over-inflated
- If hips are lower than knee level—ball is too small or under-inflated

The crunch and the extension are the two best exercises for you. The exercise ball is a wonderful piece of home equipment and will improve back health, core strength and balance.

## CRUNCH INSTRUCTION—FOR STRONG ABS

- Sit on top of ball
- Slowly walk feet forward until the ball is supporting your mid/lower back area
- Knees should be bent and feet flat on floor
- Place your arms across your chest (easier) or behind ears (harder)
- Exhale as you raise your shoulders
- Imagine peeling one vertebrae at a time from the ball
- You can stop when you feel resistance and contraction in your ab area
- As you curl up, keep the ball stable
- Inhale as you slowly lower your shoulders and head back to starting position
- Start with one set of 15 crunches at first
- Progress to two—then three sets with 45 second rests between sets

## BACK EXTENSION—FOR A STRONG LOWER BACK

- Lie facedown with ball under your hips and lower torso
- Tuck toes at the base of a wall for stability
- Place hands on shoulders (easier) or on your lower back (harder)
- Slowly roll down the ball
- Lift chest from the ball
- Bring shoulders up until body is in a straight line
- Perform same amount of repetitions as you would crunches
- Make sure head, neck, shoulders and back are in a straight line
- Keep abs contracted and never hold your breath

# Q18 How Can I Reduce the Fat Around my Hips?

There is **no such thing as spot reduction**. I repeat—the body cannot be forced to reduce fat in a specific area by exercising the muscles directly beneath the area, and yet misinformed exercisers continue to believe in the spot removal myth. The body cannot respond this way; it is not a bunch of separate parts but rather an intrinsically connected body.

## *You Can Spot Strengthen*

When you weight train your legs or hips for instance, they gain firmness from added strength. However, the bulges you wish to shrink are not made of muscle—they are made of fat, which is eliminated by losing excess body fat. To change fat to lean muscle you must create a negative caloric balance in your body and add a component of strength training to your activity.

## *Create a Negative Caloric Balance*

Overall body fat is decreased by eating fewer calories each day than you expend through movement and exercise. The familiar saying—eat less and move more is exactly what it takes to accomplish this.

## *Fat Facts*

- Men's and women's bodies deposit excess fat differently
- Women primarily store fat around the hips and buttocks
- Men store fat in the belly
- Gaining and losing fat is influenced by your age, sex and genetics
- The first place you gain fat will be the last place you lose it

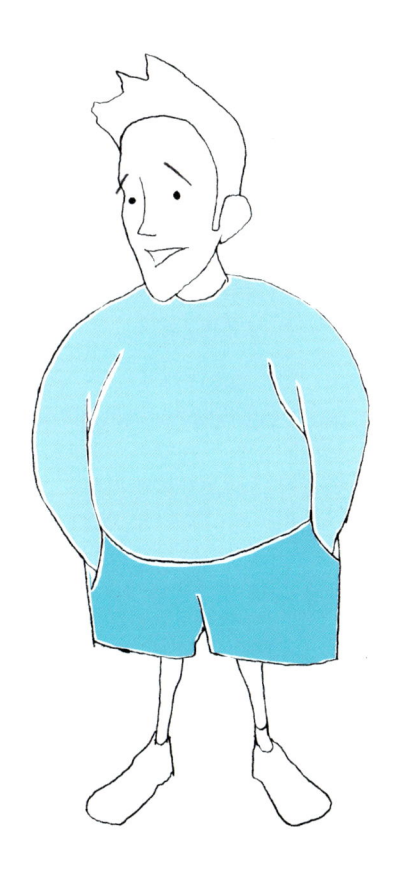

# Q19 What are the Best Exercises for Great Arms?

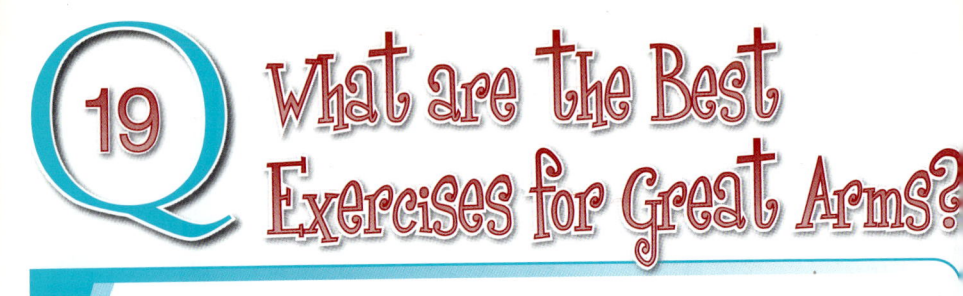

**Strong arms are attractive arms.** To have them you must spend time training the two main muscles that make up your upper arm. They are the **biceps** and the **triceps.** These muscles are what are known as opposing muscles. By this, I mean when one contracts (shortens), the other extends (lengthens) so in reality, they support each other. This is important because to achieve the best training results there must be a balance of power between the bicep and the tricep. This will not only give you great looking arms but it will also develop "joint integrity" *by keeping the shoulder and elbow joints healthy and strong.*

## *For Strong Lean Arms*

1. Weights must be heavy enough to challenge the muscles after 12 to 15 reps

2. Start with lighter dumbbells and add challenge progressively

3. Two to three sets of 12 to 15 reps will give you great results

4. Remember to warm the entire body for five or ten minutes prior to lifting

5. Finish up with a thorough upper body stretch

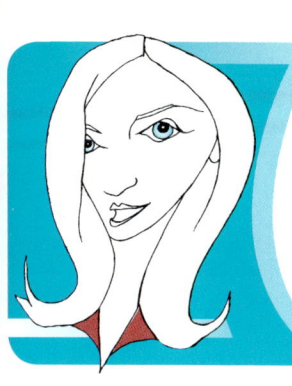

**CindySays**... *"Although the push-up primarily hits the shoulders and chest area, it is in my opinion the ultimate upper body exercise."*

## Great Arm Exercises

### ONE ARM HAMMER CURLS (BICEPS)

- Hold dumbbells and stand erect with knees slightly bent
- Keep back straight—head up
- Start with dumbbells at arms length—palms in
- Begin curl with palms in until past thighs—then turn palms up for the remainder of the curl to shoulder height
- Keep palms up while lowering until past thighs then turn palms in
- Keep upper arms close to sides and concentrate on biceps while raising and lowering weights

### TRICEP DIPS (TRICEPS, OF COURSE)

- Sit on edge of chair with feet on the floor and knees slightly bent (Tip-if too difficult just bend knees more)
- Place hands close to your body with fingers wrapped around corners of chair and thumbs facing forward
- Straighten arms by lifting buttocks up and in front of chair seat
- Slowly bend elbows as far as comfortably possible allowing hips to drop below chair seat level
- Straighten arms and lift hips back to chair seat level

## BENT-KNEE PUSH-UPS (CHEST AND SHOULDERS)

- Keep back straight and support yourself on your knees and palms
- Arms should be straight and shoulder-width apart
- Slowly lower your upper body to the floor, keeping trunk straight
- Rise back to starting position and repeat until failure

## *Food for Thought*

**Nutrition will also play a key role if you want great arms.** Muscle development and definition will always be less obvious when extra layers of fat cover it. Don't allow all your training efforts to go unnoticed by eating more calories than you are expending. A couple of percentage points of body fat can really make a noticeable difference.

# Q20 How Can I Lose Weight?

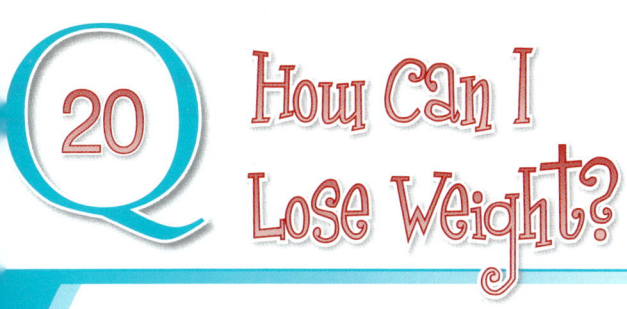

**Losing weight should be a health based decision.** If it is, then you should set your goal to lose body fat and gain lean muscle mass. Succeeding at this goal is not impossible or even complicated. It is simply the decision to make regular exercise a priority in your life and following a few basic nutritional guidelines.

## Your Weight Loss Plan

- Perform interval training rather than steady state—work at varying intensities mixing harder bouts of exercise with recovery minutes
- Eat five to six small meals each day—lean protein, fresh fruits and vegetables, whole grains and lots of water
- Diet should contain one gram of protein per pound of bodyweight for muscle health
- Lift progressively heavier weights three times a week—weights that fatigue each muscle group after twelve to fifteen reps—add more sets as your body adapts
- Rev up and revamp your training routine every four weeks to consistently challenge your body

## Q21 How Do I Get Back in Shape After Pregnancy?

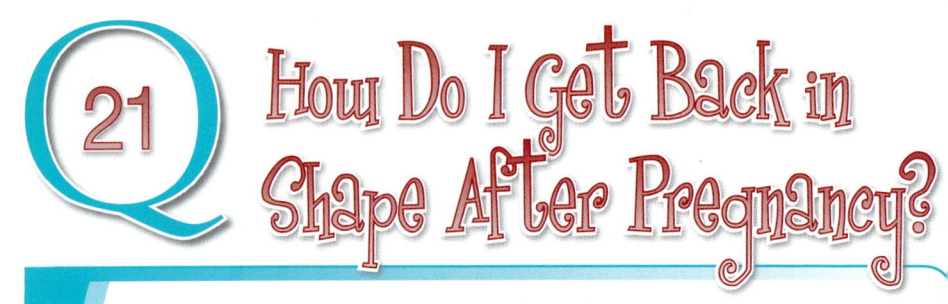

**While pregnancy and having a baby is very natural**, the changes in your body following the birth feel anything but natural. Stretched to your limit with the act of delivery and the ongoing responsibility of a new baby can leave you feeling too tired to exercise. The trick is to understand the important role your health and energy play in motherhood.

Once you are given the green light for activity, you will find that exercise actually restores your energy. Relying on the activity surrounding the care of your baby to get your firm body back will leave you frustrated. It takes time set aside for *you* and planned exercise to *build cardiovascular endurance and strengthen your muscles.* To feel comfortable in your body again, plan to address each of these.

*Biggest Challenge—Secure 30 Minutes a Day to Call Your Own—Then Use Them!*

### 30 to 60 Minutes a Day Will Give You Time For One or More of These

- Quick gym or video workout
- Refreshing power walk in your neighborhood
- Strength workout in your home away from family obligations
- Pilates class
- Yoga session

- Dance to your favorite upbeat music
- Squats and pushups
- Nice stretch and a rejuvenating bath

## *Plan Activity with Your Baby*

When weather permits, put your baby in a sturdy stroller and get moving. Make sure it has a deep seat and the seat belt attached. You should also have a safety wrist strap to prevent any kind of separation from you and the stroller. If sun is a factor, shade the baby to protect baby's skin from sunburn.

Strengthen muscles and build endurance while taking your baby for a great walk. Brisk walking is a great cardio choice but pushing and maneuvering a baby in a stroller adds the element of strength to your walk. Babies become natural progressive weights for you in your quest for fitness. They start small and grow which increases your resistance gradually and safely.

## *Be a Smart Stroller*

- Start on a smooth level sidewalk or road
- Avoid gravel surfaces and potholes as vibration is not good for baby or your joints
- Stay away from high traffic areas
- Walk with head up and a neutral spine
- Add pace and incline gradually
- Monitor your steps by wearing a pedometer
- Work toward a goal of 10,000 steps a day

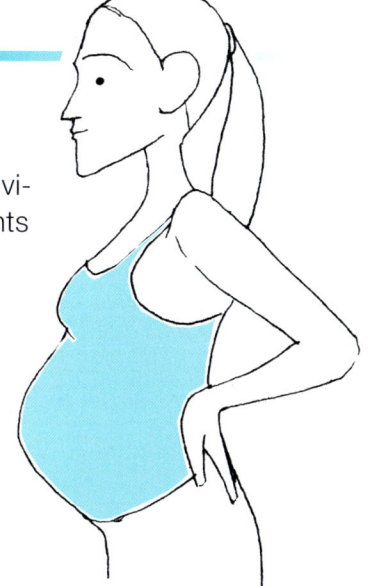

**Recognize that your nutrition and hydration** play key roles in healthy weight loss and supporting your energy requirements. Each lean protein, whole grains, and fresh fruits and vegetables and aim for 5 to 6 small meals a day rather than 3 large ones.

**Drinking eight glasses of water a day** really does help your body function optimally and can sometimes satisfy phantom hunger pains. Remember, the bottom line in losing weight is to burn more calories than you are eating. Choose a healthy food plan and keep a log of the amounts you consume each day. *Be patient and give your body the moderate exercise and the healthy foods it deserves.*

# Q22 How Do I Get Muscle Definition?

**Training a body can give you a multitude of results.** Being dedicated and diligent in the gym is wonderful but expecting to acquire a specific kind of body just because you weight train 4 days a week or even 7 days a week does not guarantee you'll get it.

Working out consistently will give you good health and a firm body, but distinct muscle definition is a result of this great physical training and a rigid nutritional plan.

The bottom line to achieve the "cut" look is that you must develop reasonably significant levels of muscle mass while at the same time reducing the amount of fat under the skin.

*I want to make clear that the pictures you see in muscle magazines aren't always as dramatic as they appear. In addition to having enhanced lighting, artificially applied tans and questionable supplementation, they are usually photographed at the culmination of a ridiculously strict, low calorie, high protein diet…void of fats and oftentimes fluids. Those preparing for a bodybuilding contest or a magazine cover will often dehydrate themselves for many hours prior to the event. This exaggerates the "cut" look. Once it is over, they rehydrate and return to a more realistic diet quickly losing the extreme muscle definition.*

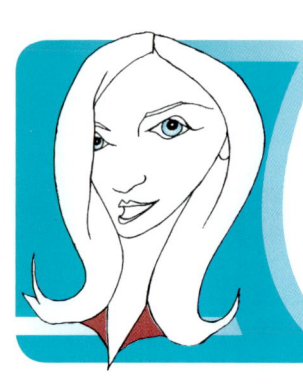

*CindySays*... *"Variety will not only reduce the possibility of overuse injury but will also keep you interested in your workouts."*

But you can reveal definition by increasing the size of the muscle and decreasing body fat. This is a good goal to set and achievable if a nutritious, low fat diet is consistently followed combined with the proper workout regimen.

## Keep This in Mind—Muscles Can Only Do Three Things

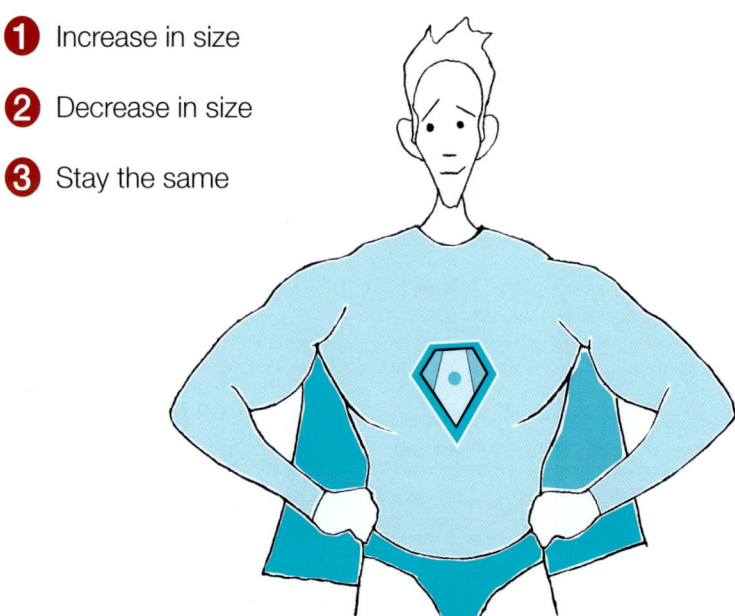

1. Increase in size
2. Decrease in size
3. Stay the same

## *Here Are A Few Tips*

- Work smart—enlist a personal trainer to offer valuable advice, evaluate your goals and make training adjustments that can make all the difference for you

- Those who achieve that "cut look" are continually challenging their muscles and staying true to good nutrition

- Muscles adapt to whatever reasonable challenge you give them in a short amount of time

- Periodic check-ups with a fitness professional can shake your workout up and add necessary challenge and increase in intensity

## Chapter 3

# THE RIGHT TYPE OF TRAINING FOR ME

**What are you preparing for physically in life?** Do you want to be a great tennis player, a cyclist, a marathon runner or perhaps you just want to be a healthy mom or dad. Chances are you are not pursuing a career in professional sports but you may possess that competitive spirit that pushes you to train hard for a recreational league just the same.

**We all want optimum health.** It's a result of an adequate combination of physical activity and quality nutrition. This should be your initial goal. From there you can fashion a training plan that matches your interests and expectations in life.

**Take racquet sports for example.**
If you are interested in becoming a great racquet ball player or tennis player, understand what demands they have on your body. For instance, these players spend a majority of time stroking the ball and moving in specific patterns. They are one-sided, repetitive sports where overuse injuries are common. Training for this type of sport should be specific to preventing tennis elbow, rotator cuff injury, back pain, and injuries to the ankle and feet through weight training and cardiovascular exercise.

**Different sports require different regimens.** This chapter will point you in the right direction and help you attain the skills you need specific to your sport of choice.

# Q23 Do I Need a Personal Trainer?

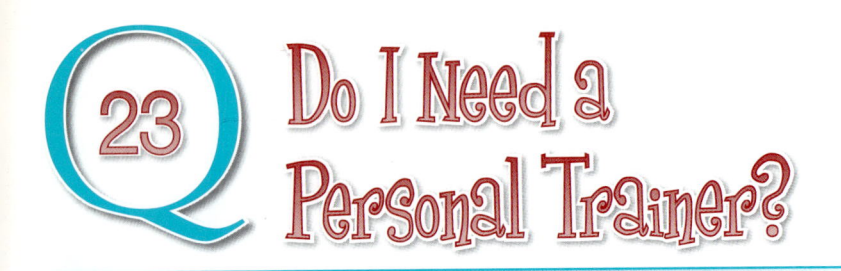

**Personal Training is one-on-one fitness instruction** created to meet the specific goals of an individual. Based on a client's goals, current level of fitness and health, and existing limitations, a training plan is designed. Typically, during regular training sessions, the personal trainer acts as a motivator while teaching proper exercise protocol, posture, and technique.

Personal training can be beneficial to anyone seeking to improve his or her fitness level and basic understanding of a healthy lifestyle. However, the act of hiring a personal trainer is not a magic bullet. It will not guarantee weight loss, better eating habits, or an enviable physique.

## Why?

- **Not all personal trainers are created equal.** They range from highly experienced people with impressive medical backgrounds to those who attended a weekend workshop. Anyone can work as a personal trainer. It is up to you to ask for credentials.

- **Personal trainers are not magicians.** Merely hiring a personal trainer and showing up at a gym will not transform your body. A personal trainer can only help you get out of a training session what you put into it.

- **Even excellent personal trainers** can only monitor what you do while they are working with you-typically no more than 3 hours per week. What you do the other 155 hours can easily prevent you from reaching your goals.

## *You May Need a Personal Trainer If*

- You have a medical condition or an injury that needs special attention
- You have no idea how to design a challenging physical program
- Your fitness plan has stalled and you are no longer making fitness strides
- You are training for a specific event and wish to enhance your performance
- You require motivation and feedback as well as someone to safely progress you

## *What to Look For If You Decide to Hire a Personal Trainer*

- Nationally recognized certification in personal training (ex)-YMCA, ACE, ACSM
- Experience or background in a medical or health related field
- Current CPR certification
- Contact information for trainer's other clients
- Thorough initial fitness assessment
- Assistance in realistic goal setting
- Thorough understanding of basic nutrition

# 24 — How Do I Become a Better Runner?

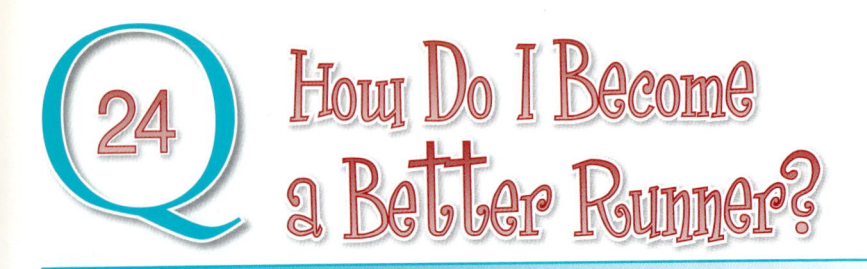

**There are several benefits** that you would receive if you were adding an aspect of strength training to your running regimen. Some runners still buy into the myth that associates strength training with big, bulky muscles. They look negatively upon anything that might result in additional weight to carry around. The fact is though—sport specific weight training does not always mean adding pounds to the runner's lean frame. What it does add to the runner is speed, power, quickness, performance, balance and injury resistance.

## Focus On

- Traditional Exercise- To strengthen the lower back and shins—two injury prone areas
- Sport Specific Exercise- imitates a runner's body movements and targets the hips, quadriceps and hamstrings
- Plyometric Exercise- improves explosive power and quickness and lengthens running stride

## Common Injuries in Running

- *Knee Injury*
- *Foot Stress Fracture*
- *Back Strain*
- *Ankle Sprain*

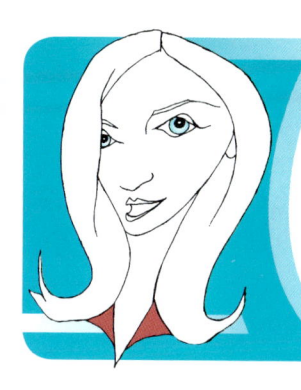

**CindySays**..."*Your chances of injury grow with every mile you log in—weight training can make the difference between running successfully for ten years and running the rest of your life.*"

## Strength Training

- Reinforces muscles, ligaments and tendons
- Helps the body resist normal stresses of repetitive running movement
- Increases joint integrity of hip, knee and ankle
- Adds bone density to prevent mechanical injury and degenerative disease
- Strengthens muscles which generate greater force and therefore greater speed
- Boosts power making running more efficient and less painful

### *A Little Weight Training Goes the Distance*

On your light running days, after a short warm up, spend 20 to 30 minutes training upper and lower body with weight that challenges you after 12 to 15 reps. Remember your muscles require a day's rest for recovery between training sessions.

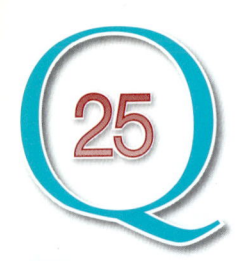

# 25 Q How Do I Train to Become a Better Skier?

**Preparation for any sport always makes good sense.** The body loses strength, flexibility and resilience as it ages if there is not at least a minimal amount of time devoted to basic body maintenance. Seven out of ten people, who end up in a hospital setting during a ski trip, do so because they weren't in ski shape. Preparation doesn't have to be exhaustive or time consuming. It simply has to be balanced and include three essential components.

## Prepare for an Active Ski Season

- *Cardiovascular Fitness*—even though skiing isn't considered an aerobic activity, it will challenge your heart over the course of a ski trip. Performance on the slopes will be enhanced if you work on *endurance training*, as you will have increased energy to keep you on the slopes rather than longing to kick back in front of the fire.

- *Strength*—skiing relies primarily on leg strength but it doesn't stop there. The entire body contributes to a skier's efficiency toward recovery when you come off the slopes. Weak muscles tax the body and make it vulnerable to injury. Those who ski without adequate *muscle strength* and endurance find themselves searching for the hot tub earlier each day.

- *Flexibility*—often overlooked but probably the most important in terms or injury prevention. Even an innocent fall can sideline you if your joints and muscles aren't pliable. Furthermore, skiing involves a great deal of abrupt trunk twisting. This sudden repetitive motion can instigate back soreness that *flexibility* can alleviate.

## Most Common Injury in Skiing

*A torn or twisted anterior cruciate ligament—ACL—is the ligament located inside the knee which bonds together the upper and lower parts of the leg and accounts for more than two-thirds of all knee injuries in skiers.*

## Making Your Training Sport Specific

- Moderate intensity aerobic activity—walk, jog, cycle, swim—to 70% of your maximum heart rate—20 to 30 minutes three times a week
- Take an interval approach to your cardiovascular workout—intense effort followed by less intense (recovery) effort
- Throw in some occasional, powerful bursts of speed
- Strength train by focusing on large muscles of legs—quadriceps, hamstrings and gluteals two to three times a week
- Squats and lunges are quite effective especially if resistance is gradually increased
- In the gym—a couple sets of leg presses, leg curls, leg extensions, hip abduction and adduction will increase lower body strength.
- Train abdominals and lower back
- Crunches and back extensions will help maintain a strong athletic stance while skiing
- Obliques work—crunching up to the opposite side—will supply power to maneuver turns with authority
- Biceps, triceps, chest, and shoulders should be strengthened with free weights or resistance machines
- Spend time stretching your back, hips and legs
- An important stretch for skiers is a T-stretch—optimally done at the end of a cardio or strength workout

## *T-stretch is the Best Stretch for Skiers*

**Lie on your back with legs pointed straight up** toward the ceiling and arms outstretched to your sides. You will resemble the letter T. While both shoulders remain in contact with the floor, slowly rotate your legs to one side toward the floor and hold for 20 to 30 seconds. Repeat on the other side and do this stretch daily to be a durable skier.

# Q26 Are Pilates and Yoga Alike?

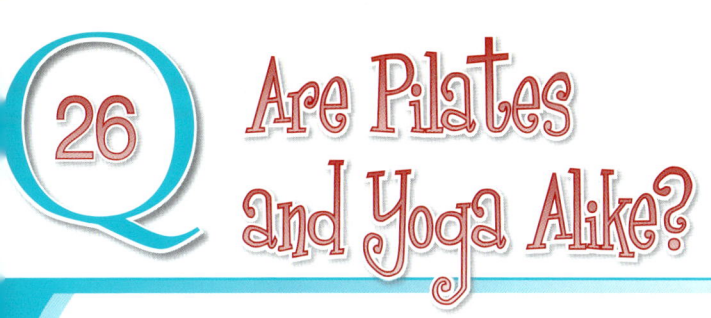

**There are definite similarities between Pilates and Yoga** as well as distinct differences. They both offer a softer form of exercise and focus on breathing and controlled movement.

## Yoga is

- Centered around Eastern idea of letting energy move through the body
- A discipline of strength and flexibility surrounded by relaxation and meditation
- Focused on helping the mind live in a state of balance

## Pilates is

- A form of exercise where physical conditioning comes first
- Like Yoga on a machine or moving yoga
- More about length, strength and stability in motion

# 27. What can Pilates Do for Me?

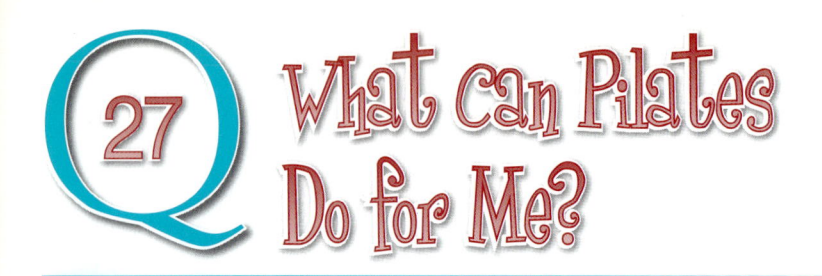

**The fitness world has embraced** the Pilates training method as a relatively *new form of exercise* even though it has been around for more than 90 years. Pilates, pronounced (pih-LAH-tees), was created as a form of rehabilitation for dancers by Joseph Pilates who lived from 1880 to 1967. Joseph Pilates was a carpenter, gymnast and a visionary. There are two ways to practice Pilates today. You can take a **mat-based class** usually held in a group setting where you will be taught any or all of the 34 basic exercises that focus on strengthening the core muscles of the body or you can take private sessions with an instructor that will most likely lead you through these exercises on **specially designed machines**.

## *The Cadillac and Reformer*

These elaborate pieces of equipment are made of cables and wood and position you so as to strengthen and lengthen your muscles in various configurations.

## *Mat Based*

All movement is performed on a mat without equipment. Exercises target your powerhouse muscles -- abs, lower back, thighs, and buttocks— and focus on proper alignment and elongation of the musculature.

## Good News if You are Looking for Kinder and Gentler

**Pilates is low to non-impact.** Nothing is forced or repetitive and emphasis is placed on form rather than intensity. It can be used as rehabilitative training therefore, most people are good candidates except those who are in a state of fragility. It is also a solution to exercisers facing training boredom.

## Don't Look to Pilates for Weight Loss

**It is not considered a means to lose weight.** While you will most likely strengthen your body and gain many health benefits such as joint mobility, decreased stress and improved circulation, you will need to incorporate cardiovascular training for a complete workout. Also, if you like to master things quickly, this may not be the workout for you. Like dance, yoga and martial arts, Pilates is a long-term evolutionary practice.

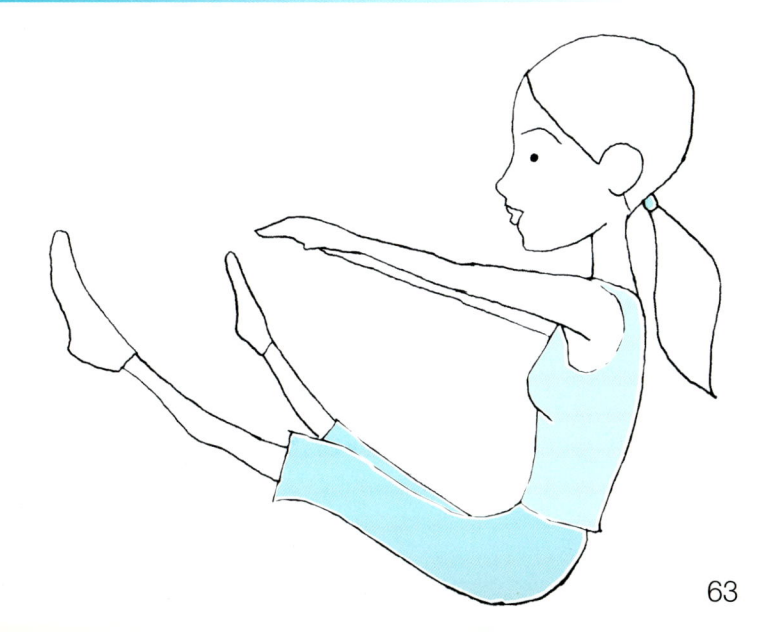

# Q28. How Do I Know if I Have a Bad Personal Trainer?

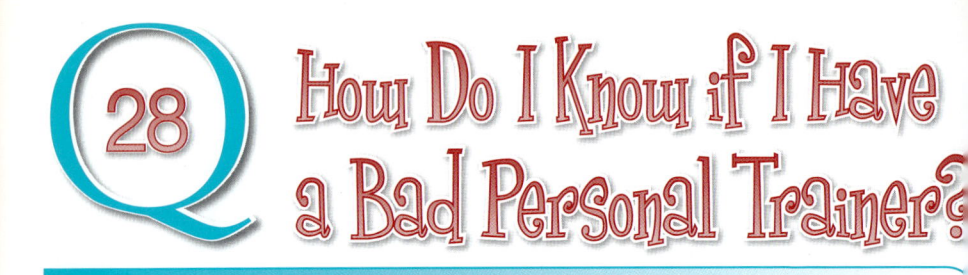

**The service of a personal trainer** provides you with information, motivation and the most efficient way to improve your fitness level. The personal trainer should be all about **YOU** and **YOUR GOALS**!

## You May Have a BAD Personal Trainer if He or She:

- Is not *nationally* certified with current CPR
- Has not completed a thorough *assessment* prior to designing your program
- Shows up *late* or unprepared for your session
- Fails to warm you up with *dynamic* movement
- Stretches you *before* your workout
- Uses cardiovascular equipment as a warm up or for more than 5 minutes
    - ✓ Exception: GOOD trainers may use cardio machines for more intense interval training bouts for an aerobic response
- Has not provided you with a *plan* for training independently
- Spends more than 15 minutes of your workout on *unstable devices* such as
    - ✓ BOSU
    - ✓ Exercise Ball
    - ✓ Wobble Board

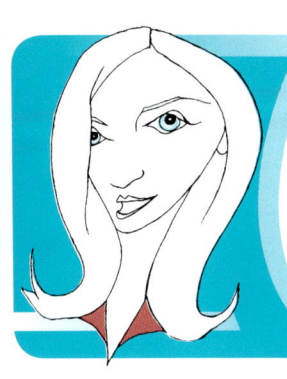

**CindySays**..."*If you are contracting a personal trainer with these qualities, you are probably not making progress. If you are making progress in spite of this, you probably don't need a personal trainer!*"

- Has not changed your training regimen in *4 weeks*
- Changes your workout *every* time with little structure
- Is not giving you his or her *undivided attention*
    - ✓ He leaves you to answer someone's questions/to demonstrate an exercise
- Instructs you to do more than 10 to 15 minutes of *core training*
- Is not monitoring your *form and technique* on every repetition performed
- Is unable to *modify* or choose alternative exercises according to your limitations
- Is more focused on *body weight* rather than body fat (composition)
- Does not monitor *body composition* changes on a regular basis
- Is not motivating you or seems *disconnected* during training
- Fails to give *posture cues* as you exercise
- Designs programs that are either *unchallenging* or *too challenging*
- Is unable to answer *fundamental* questions on exercise and nutrition
- Attempts to prescribe exercise and/or nutritional advice *beyond his scope* of expertise and education
- Is unable to give you *clear reasons* to justify why he is prescribing a specific training regimen for you

- Has not designed your program around the *six basic human movements*
    - ✓ Push
    - ✓ Pull
    - ✓ Lunge
    - ✓ Squat
    - ✓ Bend
    - ✓ Twist
- Spends more than 20% of your session on *resistance machines* rather than on free weights and/or pulleys
- Does not correct muscle imbalances through *proper stretching*
- Designs an exercise program that closely resembles a *circus act*
- Builds in either *too much* or *too little* recovery time between strength training movements to facilitate maximal benefit
- Your trainer fails to *monitor recovery* time
- Is not a good role model …does not *"walk the walk"*

## Q29 Am I a Bad Personal Training Client?

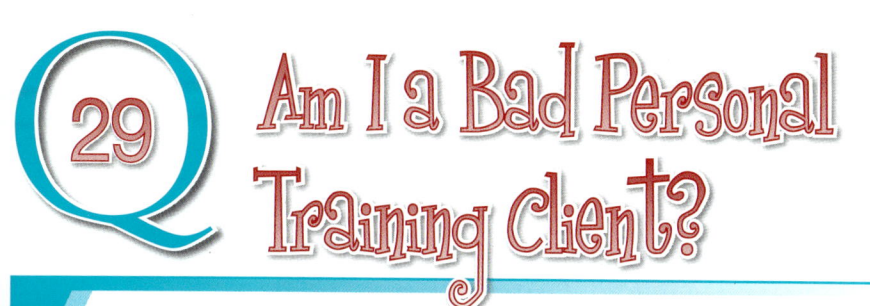

**If your working with a trainer and not achieving your fitness goals,** consider the possibility the one sabotaging your progress just might be **YOU**. That's right—the results you get from the act of hiring and paying for personal training is directly linked to your commitment and performance. Here is a checklist for you to determine whether you might be a bad personal training client.

### You Might Be a Bad Personal Training Client if You:

- Expect the trainer to help you reach unrealistic goals
- Arrive late for your personal training appointments
- Show up poorly prepared to expend energy
- Didn't get adequate rest the night before
- Lack focus during the workout
- Haven't consumed nutritious calories 1½ to 2 hours prior to your workout
- Aren't sufficiently hydrated with fluids/water
- Routinely complain about the exercises your trainer asks you to do—*the exception here is that if something hurts you should tell your trainer*

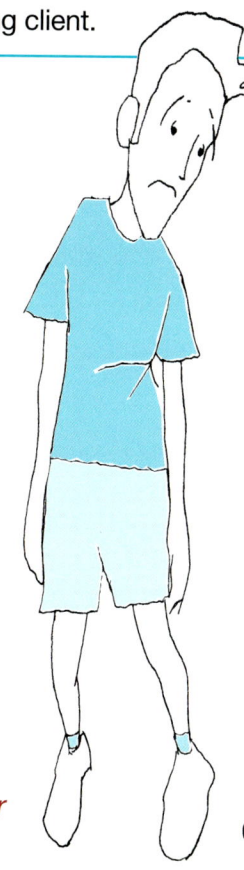

- Cancel appointments frequently
- Attempt to work out when you are sick
- Fail to disclose unhealthy lifestyle habits—such as smoking, bulimia, drug use
- Aren't following the trainer's directives with regard to physical activity and nutrition apart from session
- Won't keep a dietary log if requested to or keep an inaccurate log
- Consume empty calories—too much alcohol, sweets, fried foods, etc
- Eat too little
- Exercise only while working with the trainer
- Exaggerate independent physical activity claims
- Lack a proactive spirit—uninterested in the *how's* and *why's* of your personal program
- Believe that just "showing up"—*not giving 100%* –for your session will be productive
- Come to workout in unsupportive or inappropriate footwear
- Appeal for longer recovery periods during your training session
- Postpone scheduled body composition measurements
- Basically lack an ongoing commitment

**Many dedicated personal trainers reach a frustrating end** with clients who believe the act of hiring a trainer will automatically be a magic bullet. If you are a client unable to dedicate the energy or unwilling to comply with the demands/sacrifices of the trainer's plan, you will have difficulty reaching your fitness goals.

**Realizing fitness goals is not easy for anyone.** We all fall off the health wagon now and again. Buying into the myth that a personal trainer can counteract poor lifestyle choices and habits is a foolish investment. It requires a respectful commitment from you and your personal trainer in order to see the results you both desire.

# Q30 What is Isometric Exercise?

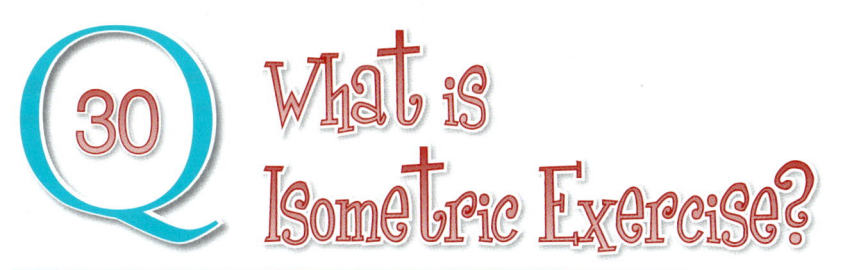

**Isometric exercise is a type of exercise** that creates resistance in the muscle *without movement in the muscle.* Tension is created and maintained while holding the muscle in a stationary position for a set count.

## Three Things Can Occur When a Muscle is Stimulated

- The muscle becomes shorter *(concentric exercise)*
- The muscle becomes longer *(eccentric exercise)*
- The muscles remains the same length *(isometric exercise)*

Isometric exercise is used primarily for those people who may be rehabilitating from an injury that has caused them to either temporarily or permanently lose range of motion in the joint. However, unless this is the case, there are better ways to train the muscle. Stronger muscles and joints are acquired by working the muscle with progressive resistance and repetition through their entire range of motion.

Isometric exercises in conjunction with weight training add variety and reach muscle fatigue. This is done by holding the tension at the peak of the contraction at the end of a set.

# Q31 How Can I Do Step Aerobics Safely?

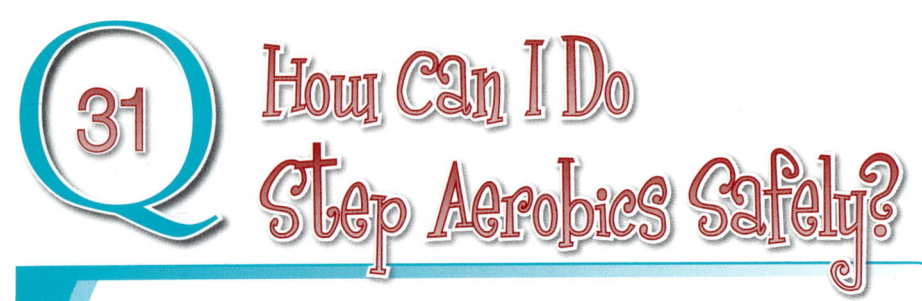

**Step aerobics or step training,** born in the eighties, is a versatile form of low impact exercise when performed properly. It is safe for the novice and can be challenging to the veteran exerciser.

There are considerations with regard to safety when choosing step aerobics as a primary form of cardiovascular exercise—step height, stepping speed and type of steps performed.

## Safety Guidelines

- People with chronic knee problems need physician's approval before stepping
- The newer you are to step the lower the height of your step should be
- Step height should never cause the knee joint to flex more than 90 degrees
- Always step up with entire foot on the step platform-do not let heel hang off edge
- Step softly so that it remains a low-impact activity
- Never step more than one shoe length away from step to protect your Achilles tendon
- Limit *repeaters* to five consecutive—*non-weight-bearing leg repeats movement*
- Limit *propulsion* steps to one minute—*both feet are off the floor at same time*

- Change lead leg after no more than one minute
- Master footwork before adding upper body movement
- Step music faster than 122 beats per minute is risky and not recommended

## You Can Even Do it Without the Step

**One of the great aspects of step training is** that steps prompted by the instructor can be duplicated on the floor without using the step which will instantly lower your intensity and simplify confusing movement on the step. This also allows progression and adaptation. Step has proven to be one of the safest ways to burn calories and build lower body strength when instructors and participants abide by safety guidelines.

# Q32 What is Functional Training?

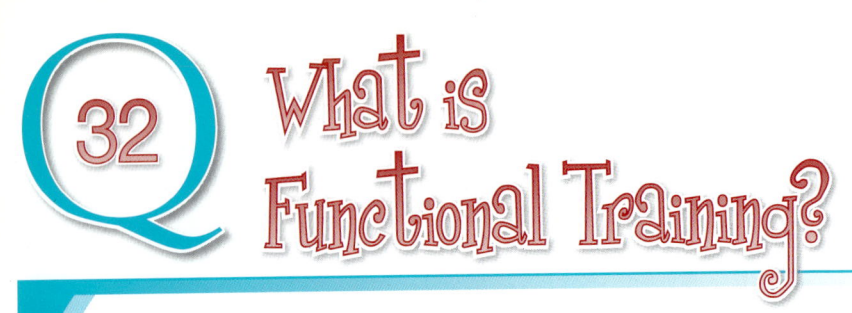

**A fitness industry buzz-word,** functional training is defined as *the integration of balance and intrinsic muscular stability during the exertion of muscular force.*

Integration is the key word. Before *functional training* became popular, people went into gyms and climbed onto resistance training machines and *isolated* muscles as they worked out. They would work each particular muscle such as the biceps before they moved to a different machine to work the triceps, hamstrings or the quadriceps.

In functional training, we don't isolate muscles—we integrate—by recruiting or working several muscles simultaneously. An example of this would be a pull-up exercise which works the *biceps, abdominals, lower back, shoulders and lats* all at the same time.

## Functional Training

- Is multi-dimensional, multi-joint and closely resembles natural movement
- Encourages use of free weights and stabilizing equipment such as balance balls
- Gets people off health club machines
- Receives no external support for balance or strength
- Forces the body to continually maintain equilibrium

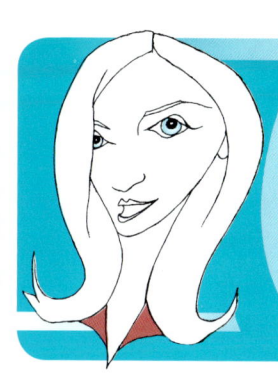

***CindySays***... *"Functional training may be difficult for beginners who may be better off starting on machines which guide the body safely through a proper range of motion and form."*

- A great way to increase overall strength and conditioning
- Helps improve ease and performance of daily activities and sports
- Very time efficient as by definition it works many muscles simultaneously

# Q33 How Do I Get Better at Racquet Sports?

**Racquet sports place great physical demands on your body.** Many recreational players spend a majority of time on the courts stroking the ball and practicing serves and very little time creating a durable body that will withstand the wear and tear of these lifetime sports. Often, it is not until the body breaks down that conditioning is considered necessary. Stay ahead of the game by training smart.

## Focus On

*Cardiovascular Conditioning*—simulate racquet sport movement as part of training

*Foot Speed*—gets you to the ball in time to be balanced and ready to swing your racquet

*Quickness*—ability to change direction while in motion or from starting position

*Muscle Endurance*—staying power

*Explosive Strength*—for speed and quickness

*Balance of Strength*—counterbalancing repetitive one-sided sport and injury prevention

## Common Overuse Injuries in Racquet Sports

- Tennis Elbow
- Shoulder
- Back Strain
- Ankle Sprain

## Making Your Training Sport Specific

- Simulate authentic sport movements as part of your cardiovascular work. *Short sprints, back-peddling, cross-over steps and shuffling side to side* will supply you with adequate conditioning while preparing your body to move with more grace and efficiency around the court.

- Strength is the foundation of speed and quickness. Incorporate explosive strength training and plyometrics into your workouts. *Leaping, bounding and training with medicine balls and resistance bands* are effective ways to train.

- Strengthen and stabilize all areas of the shoulder to absorb the pounding of the ball. *Mimic your racquet sport movements with light resistance* to increase muscle resiliency and neuromuscular coordination.

- Core muscles—abdominal and lower back—link the upper and lower extremities and are essential in maintaining the integrity of a strong body. *Rotate side to side as you would for a forehand and backhand using a medicine ball* to develop strength in these areas.

Specific training for racquet sports is the most efficient way to improve your game. General weight training will improve the strength and endurance of your muscles. However, conditioning with a focus on the muscles that you rely on will take you a step further—giving you a stronger body and make you a more competitive player.

# Q34 How Do I Train for Speed and Quickness?

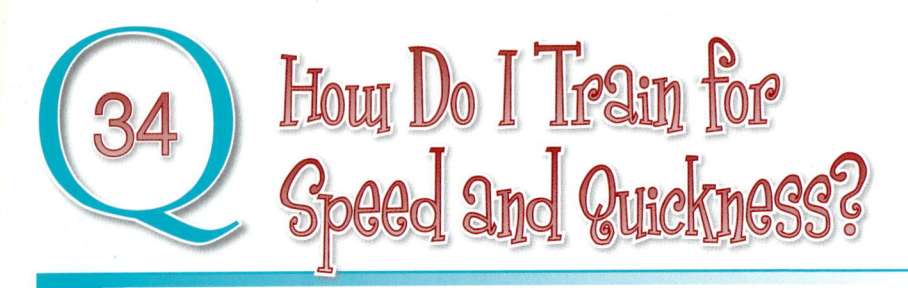

**First understand there is a difference between speed and quickness.** Although you may hear these words synonymously, training for them is not the same.

Speed is how fast you can go from point A to point B. Quickness on the other hand, relies on how quickly your neuromuscular system responds to your brain asking it to move or how quickly your muscles react and contract. ***Think of quickness as the initial part of speed.***

Coaches look for athletes with quickness because it encompasses more than speed. It is based on the brain's reaction time and instantaneous recruitment of the body's motor units to make muscles move. Quickness is somewhat determined by heredity but can be improved with training.

## Maximize Your Ability to React Quickly

- Train hips and abdominals which control your running potential
- Train with Plyometric movements to improve explosiveness
- Train to be flexible to unleash your power and avoid injury
- Although you are training via physical movement…you are essentially training your nervous system to send messages to your muscles. This neural training is what will improve quickness. Repeated rehearsals of these proper movements will result in muscles receiving the mes-

sage faster than before. Believe it or not, muscles have memory and the more you practice a movement…*for example, bursting out of the blocks at the start of a 40 yard dash*…the quicker you will become. Keep in mind that your practice form must be perfect otherwise your muscles will remember and therefore, repeat flawed form.

## Useful Tools for Developing Quickness

- Agility ladders
- Plyo boxes
- Resistance equipment such as parachutes or power sleds
- Hurdles
- Jump Rope
- Cones

Quickness is a valuable element in optimum athletic performance. Improving overall strength and conditioning is the first important step toward maximizing your potential quickness.

# Q35 How Do I Train to Be a Better Cyclist?

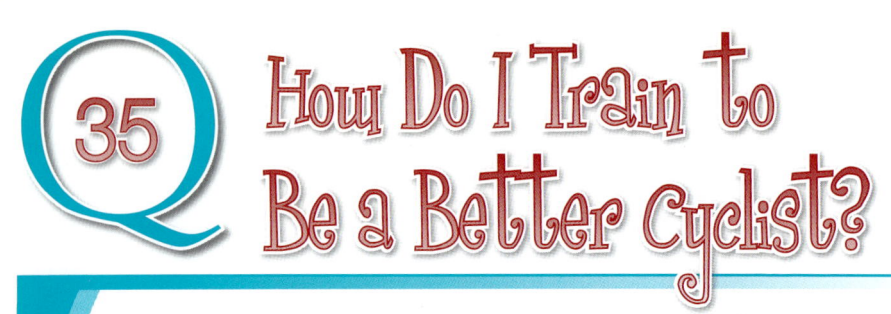

**A rider who is in better shape** will ride more efficiently for longer periods at any speed. To accomplish this, training must be year round and go beyond the confines of a bike.

Cross training will address overall fitness and prevent burnout from boredom. Stationary cycling can be quite monotonous while looking at the same four walls.

## Focus On

- *Cross-training cardio work*—*cross-country skiing, swimming, in-line skating*
- *Weight training*—*higher weights and fewer reps* during off-season and *lower weights and more reps* just before and during cycling season
- *Flexibility*—because cycling freezes posture for long periods of time, it is essential to spend time on *range of motion and flexibility.*
- *Technique*—stationary cycling with *one-legged spinning* to be a better peddler and improve riding technique

## Weight Training Helps in Sprints and Jumps

- Upper body strength allows maximum power from the legs around the pedal. It also minimizes the amount of inefficient rocking in the shoulders during sprints and hill climbs.

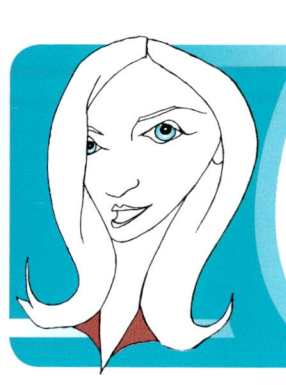

***CindySays...****"Remember to build in recovery days. One day a week off the bike and easy spin days will make you a better cyclist."*

- Muscle strength in the lower body can enable a cyclist to ride up a hill rather than walk it.
- A strong body adds injury prevention to the rider's body for inevitable falls along the way.
- Muscles endurance reduces fatigue and wear and tear on the body and aids in recovery after a difficult ride.

# 36. Can I Add Too Much Muscle to my Body?

Just as some are obsessed with losing weight—***a disorder known as anorexia***—and venture into habits such as excessive calorie restriction and/or bulimia, there are those—6% of all men who weight train—who are on the opposite end of the continuum who are obsessed with gaining weight and building muscle—***a disorder known as Megarexia.*** Either end of this spectrum is extremely detrimental to good health.

Much like the anorexic, the megarexic has a distorted perception of their body and classified as a ***dysmorphic or obsessive-compulsive disorder.*** It is not uncommon for people to feel insecure about their appearance—this is what motivates some of us to start eating healthier and exercising regularly.

Unfortunately, for some, these feelings of inadequacy become so overwhelming that muscle building becomes their mission in life. When conventional weight training doesn't yield the results they crave, they resort to compulsive behaviors in order to gain bulging stomach muscles, huge backs and prominent biceps.

## Signs of Unhealthy Behavior

- Sacrifice relationships, job or school responsibilities in order to meet rigid exercise routines
- May weight train even while injured
- Resort to unhealthy supplements and/or steroids despite the risks

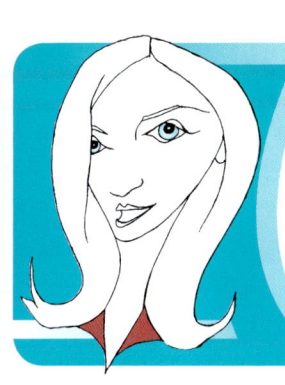

***CindySays***..."*When physical training dominates and interferes with the enjoyment of life, seek counsel with a therapist who specializes in body image.*"

- Perceive themselves as having insufficient muscularity
- Feel they are a mere shadow of the physical bodies they inhabit
- Compulsive mirror checkers—up to twelve times a day
- Spend up to six hours a day training with weights

# Q37 How Can I Improve My Balance?

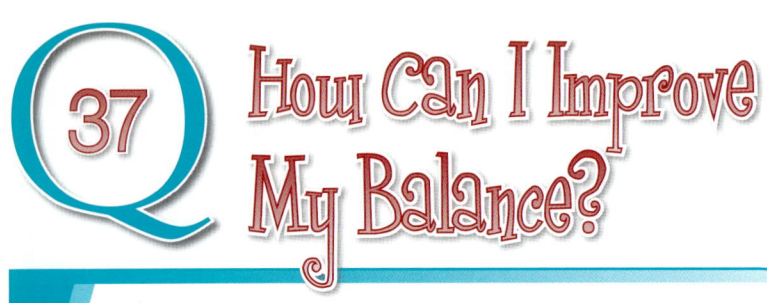

We know cardiovascular conditioning, strength training and flexibility key components of fitness. However, balance or kinesthetic awareness is gaining respect among people seriously pursuing fitness. *Balance is the ability to find and maintain equilibrium while in a stationary position or during movement.*

Balance is the foundation of all movement and should be respected as a vital part of a healthy life. From birth we struggle to achieve balance and throughout life it is a skill we must continue to work on. Everyone—from the newest exerciser to the elite athlete benefits from balance training. It is as necessary for the gymnast as it is for the person who unsuspectingly steps from a curb in the dark.

## Tools To Enhance Balance Performance

- Balance Beam on the Floor
- Large Balance Ball
- Foam Roller
- Wobble Board
- Bosu Ball

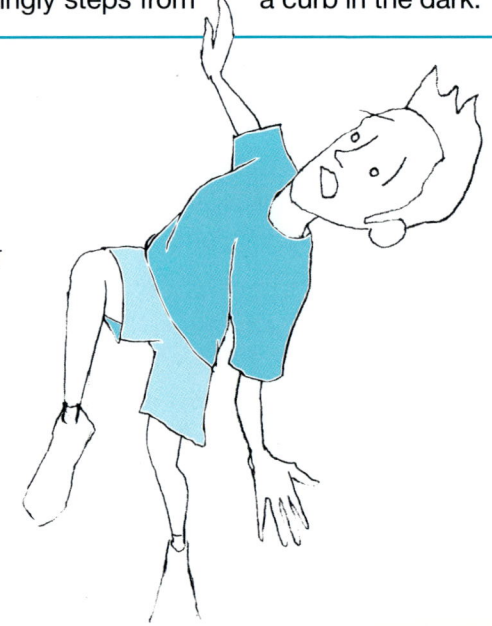

## Test Your Balance

**This test is also a balance training exercise.** Stand on one foot, reach forward to touch the floor in front of you then resume a standing position on the same foot.

- This Exercise Can Be Progressed In Many Different Ways
- Stand on one foot and add small movements with the lifted leg
- Close one eye or both as you stand on one foot
- Catch a ball as you balance on one foot
- Practice dipping down and raising up while on one foot

## Other Forms Of Exercise To Improve Balance

- Tai Chi-emphasizes precise, graceful body movements
- Step movement which demands balance in motion
- Pilates which trains the body's core musculature
- Yoga which strengthens the body while holding various postures

## Chapter 4

# Injury, Illness and Limitation

**What prevents you from participating in regular exercise?** Is it too difficult due to a limitation—do you finish your activity in pain because of the remnants of an old injury—do you anticipate discomfort when planning to exercise—are you unsure about what type of activity is safe for you? You are not alone. Most everyone has an affliction/limitation of one kind or another—some are more severe than others, and ALL can create roadblocks to your good health.

**Your roadblock could be everyday aches and pains;** chronic debilitating pain; de-conditioned body stemming from too many poor lifestyle choices; a medical condition that limits activity; or worn or torn joints and ligaments from injury or accident.

**Perhaps the reason you avoid activity** isn't pain or discomfort but rather that you lack positive and enjoyable exercise experiences. Or maybe, you like it, but need a plan of action—some direction to enable you to feel good not only, during your workout, but more importantly, after your workout.

**This chapter examines the many barriers** responsible for years of debilitating detours. Whether it is pain, disease, lack of mobility or just a complete dislike of exercise and sweat, this chapter will offer you alternative pathways capable of leading you to a place where you can live healthier. It offers advice based on modification and directs you to areas of activity that work for you.

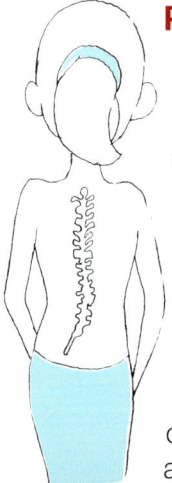

# Q38 What Causes Shin Splints?

**Shin splints**—media tibial stress syndrome—is a "catch all" term for a wide array of conditions such as muscle inflammation, tendonitis, periostitis (a muscle to bone inflammation), compartment syndromes and stress fractures.

The *tibia* is the larger of the two bones between your ankle and knee. You experience pain when tiny fibers of the membrane that attach muscles to your tibia become irritated and inflamed.

## Causes of Shin Splints

- Failing to progress exercise gradually - too much, too soon, too hard
- Over-doing athletic activities
- Participating in sports with a great deal of abrupt stops
- Running down hill
- Lack of proper warm-up
- Too little post exercise stretching
- Unsupportive shoes
- Improper body mechanics—bad form

If you have ever had shin splints, you will want to know how to prevent them from reoccurring in addition to a thorough warm up and post stretch.

## Pain Prevention Tips

- **Wear proper footwear**—understand different forms of activity require different shoes—extra pair of socks may help too
- **Check shoes for mileage**—good for about 400 miles—may look good on the outside but shock absorption is gone from the inside
- **Run or walk on the most forgiving surfaces you can find**—asphalt is better than cement—dirt is better than asphalt—grass is better than dirt
- **Avoid long distance track work with tight turns**—too stressful on inside of lower legs
- **Pay attention to mechanics**—land first on heel—roll into ball of foot—push off through the toes—*NEVER land flat-footed!*
- **Strengthen lower leg muscles**—shins, calves, ankles with weighted toe raises

## Already got them—Help!

- Alleviate stress by minimizing frequency, intensity or time of activity
- Change your activity altogether—swim or concentrate on upper body
- Massage affected area often with ice to reduce pain and inflammation

If you suspect you have shin splints, see a sports medicine physician for an accurate diagnosis—especially if you have increasing pain during workouts or numbness and/or tingling of your ankle or foot.

# Q39 How Do I Prevent Backaches?

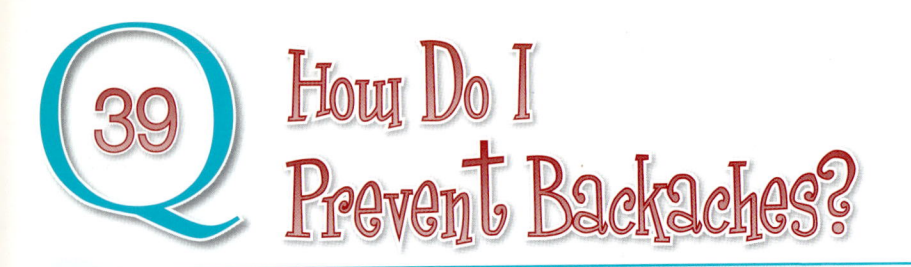

**Whether the pain is a dull aching annoyance** or piercing and unbearable, back pain gets your attention. Chronic back pain shows up in many forms and varies for each person. The same strain can present itself with muscle spasms or tenderness in one person and incapacitate another person with radiating pain to other parts of the body.

**By the time we reach adulthood,** most of us have experienced a back problem of one kind or another. Those who have, understand how seriously back pain affects our ability to work, play, sleep, and move through our every day life.

## Causes

- Injury
- Repetitive occupations such as factory work, nursing, construction
- Occupations in a seated position such as office work, truck driver
- Occupations in a standing position such as hairdresser, retail sales
- Movement that involves heavy lifting or bending and twisting motion

### Keep in Mind

Jobs requiring physical work cannot replace the need for regular exercise. Instead you must keep your body flexible and strong so the physical strain of your work has a minimized impact on your body.

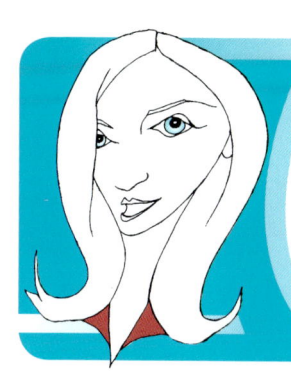

***CindySays***... *"Consider taking a gentle or beginner yoga class if you are dealing with back pain. It can be a great way to alleviate discomfort by developing strong and flexible body."*

## *Preventative Exercise*

- Cardiovascular for weight management, strong heart and lungs and energy
- Strength training including upper back, lower back, and abdominals
- Stretching exercises that focus on the soft tissues in the back and around the spine
- Range of motion exercise to keep the entire body flexible
- Practice good posture and take frequent breaks from sitting or standing too long

*All exercise for the back should be controlled, gradual, and progressive.* The goal is to have a flexible spine and to improve general body strength and muscle balance. Muscle weakness, stiffness, and imbalance are the three major contributors to back pain.

*Your spine needs to be activated regularly* to prevent undue stress to your back when you find yourself in a compromised posture with an excessive workload. Achieving a strong and flexible back is not about simply doing back exercises. It is about maintaining strong muscles from the neck down. Your back is your stabilizer and if your legs or arms are not capable of meeting the demands you place on them, your back will take up the slack. Continually placing this type of exertion on your spine will eventually show up in the way of back pain or injury.

## Stretch Your Hamstrings

**The hamstring muscles play a key role in low back pain**, as those who have low back pain tend to have tight hamstrings, and people with tight hamstrings tend to have low back pain. Hamstring tightness limits motion in the pelvis and can place it in a position that increases stress across the low back.

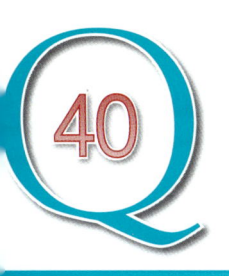

# Q40 What Exercise is Helpful for Scoliosis?

**Scoliosis is a musculoskeletal disorder** noted by a sideways or lateral curvature of the spine or backbone. Provided the curvature of the spine is less than 20 degrees, any sport or recreational activity will minimize any potential decrease in function over time. Remaining physically fit is important. You should choose exercises that build bone density, muscle strength, and flexibility.

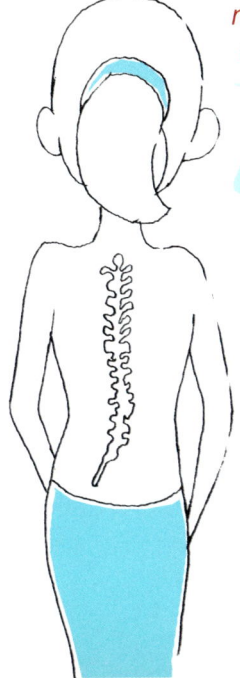

*For anyone exercising with scoliosis, postural alignment is a critical concern and should be considered a priority.*

## Posture and Performance Points

1. Pilates and yoga will address postural imbalances
2. Focus on balance of muscle in terms of strength and flexibility
3. A large exercise ball is a valuable tool to stretch and strengthen core and back
4. Stay active and focus on consistent mobility
5. Consult with a physical therapist for a postural assessment

# Q41 I Have Plantar Fasciitis What can I Do?

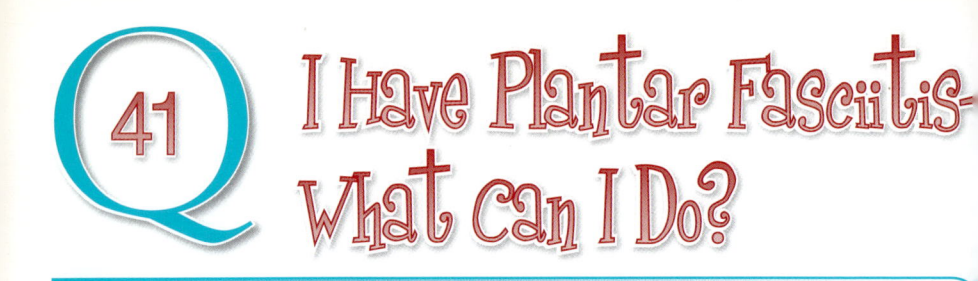

**Plantar Fasciitis**—*inflamed arch*—is quite painful, especially when you first get out of bed. You can probably draw a straight line through the length of your foot where it hurts. This is the thick fibrous band of tissue you call the arch that connects your heel to your toes.

## Causes of Plantar Fasciitis

- Poorly fitted shoes
- Standing on your feet for extended periods of time
- Misaligned walking mechanics

## Pain Prevention Tips

- Your shoe size changes with age and weight—don't assume you still wear the same size—get measured by a foot specialist if in doubt
- Minimize standing or stressing the feet
- Cushioned gel inserts may reduce pressure and trauma to arch
- Control your weight with exercise like swimming or cycling
- Have your foot alignment checked by a professional—Podiatrists can custom make an orthotic (shoe insert) to correct a rolling in or rolling out of the foot
- Avoid activity that causes pain to the arch

## *Already got them—Help!*

- Ice massage the length of your arch several minutes three times a day
- Gentle stretching—pull back on your toes and ball of your foot and hold for 20 seconds—repeat five to ten times
- Wear cushioned gel inserts to reduce stress—*remember—they will not fix a misalignment problem if you are coming in contact with the ground improperly*
- See a foot specialist if pain persists

# Q42 My Knees Hurt – How Can I Stay Active?

**There are many reasons for pain in the knees.** Sadly, it is a major reason for inactivity and weight gain due to the extreme discomfort during movement.

## Causes of Knee Pain

- *Osteoarthritis*—joint degeneration *(MOST COMMON)*
- *Injury or trauma*—ligament and tendon tears
- *Obesity*—puts constant undue stress on knee joint
- *Bursitis*—most common in people who kneel for extended periods of time
- *Osgood-Schlatter Disease*—irritation of growth plate that affects adolescents
- *Chondromalacia Patella*—due to softening of the cartilage

Because knee pain tends to make people less and less active most of these conditions progressively worsen. Inactivity is not the answer. Being sedentary is far more detrimental and finding the appropriate tolerable movement is the key. Activity in moderation keeps your cardiovascular system fit, encourages flexibility, helps you maintain a healthy body weight, decreases pain and gives you a feeling of well being.

Low impact activity at a moderate pace is what your body requires. Movement that is performed after slowly warming up the body and followed with range-of-motion stretches will keep the muscles and tendons that power the knee joint strong and flexible.

Physical therapy is an important aspect of treatment for knee pain. Depending upon the severity and cause, a physical therapist can design a reasonable exercise plan that will increase strength, regain mobility, and improve function.

## Appropriate Types of Exercise

- Swimming and water walking—*(MOST TOLERABLE)*
- Stationary cycling
- Pilates
- Yoga
- Tai Chi

Weight management should be a priority when dealing with knee pain. Nutrition and portion control combined with appropriate activity can manage weight and lessen the trauma to the knee.

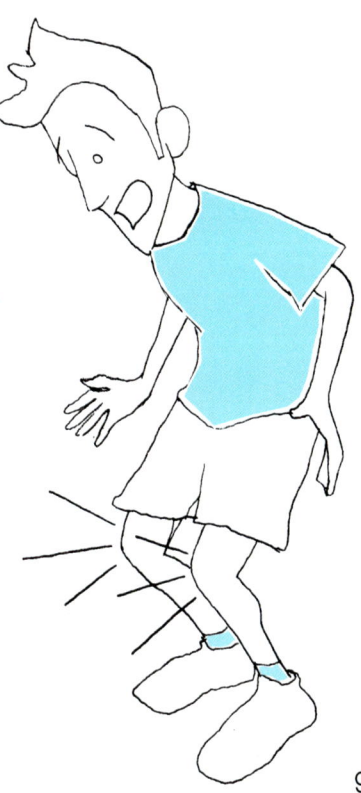

# Q43 I Have Osteoporosis— Can Exercise Help?

**Osteoporosis** is a degenerative bone disease sometimes referred to as the "silent disease" because it is often not diagnosed until there is a fracture. Men and women build bone density and generally reach peak bone density levels in their early thirties. From that point on, unless aggressively promoted and maintained through diet and exercise, bone mass declines. Sedentary individuals lose bone mass at a rapid rate as opposed to active individuals.

## Prevention Within Our Control

- Amount of dietary calcium and vitamin D intake
- Frequency and intensity of weight-bearing exercise
- Smoking

## Prevention Beyond Our Control

- Gender-Females have a greater risk
- Race-Fair skinned persons have a greater risk
- Age-Risk increases as we age

Post-menopausal females who are fair skinned are at greatest risk for osteoporosis. However, anyone, including men, can be at risk. Prevention is the key in dealing with this.

**Weight-bearing exercise is extremely valuable** because it stresses the muscles and, therefore, the bone. When we lift weights, walk briskly, dance, climb stairs, mow grass, practice martial arts, take a land aerobics class, ski, skate, play sports or hike, we are doing weight-bearing exercise.

**These activities stress our muscles and pull against our bones,** forcing them to react. Our bones respond by becoming denser and stronger.

## We Often Overlook the Upper Body

Most activities, such as walking, are adequate for the lower body. *Walking will not build bone density in the shoulder, arm or wrist, and the wrist is one of the most common sites of fracture in older adults.* To maintain bone mass in the upper body, we must stress our arms, shoulders and wrists by lifting weights, or working against resistance.

## Examples of Weight-Bearing Exercise for Upper Body

- Push-ups
- Free-weight work
- Heavy gardening
- Resistance bands and machines

## Building Bone Density in Older Adults

- 30 minutes of upper and lower body weight-bearing exercise three to four times a week
- Limit red meat, alcohol, caffeine, and soft drinks

- 800 mg. calcium dairy products and dark green leafy vegetables
- 400 to 800 IU vitamin D to aid absorption of calcium
- Consult your physician about medication to rebuild bone density

Weight-training remains a key factor when it comes to prevention of osteoporosis. Once a fracture occurs, the individual is likely to be more sedentary, often proliferating the disease. The harder we work our bones the stronger they become.

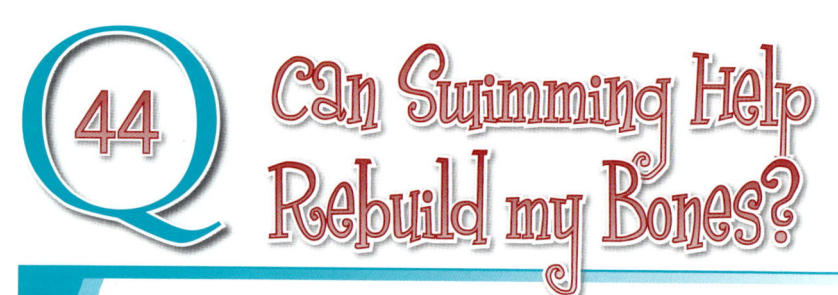

## Q44 Can Swimming Help Rebuild my Bones?

***Unfortunately, swimming is not a weight-bearing form of exercise.*** However, for many people who have severe osteoporosis and are unable to tolerate land activities, it can be a great alternative. While it won't stimulate bone development, it will strengthen muscle which supports the bone as well as increase flexibility in and around the joints which may alleviate some pain associated with this disease. Swimming and water aerobics will also improve the cardiovascular system and give you a better sense of well being.

# Q45 How Can I Stay Active with Osteoarthritis?

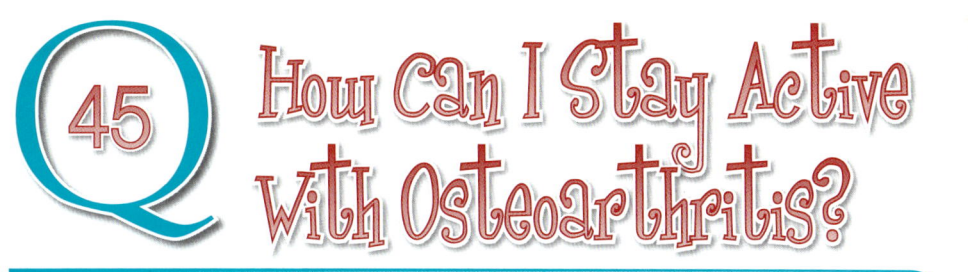

**We all come to "moments of truth"** with our bodies. Whether it is wear and tear, abuse, accident, illness, or simply age, oftentimes, our heart is more durable than the physical structure that houses it. In fact, few elude limitation altogether while pursuing active lifestyles. This is not a time to lament what you cannot do—rather; it is the time to be open to other avenues of exercise.

**Osteoarthritis is the "wear and tear"** variety of arthritis. Joints affected by osteoarthritis have little or no cartilage left for protection. This causes friction as the bones rub against one another. It is painful and results in swelling and reduced freedom of motion. If care is not taken, damage to the joint will continue and can deteriorate enough to become deformed.

## *There Are Some Preventive Measures to Heed*

- Stay close to your ideal weight
- Consume foods rich in Calcium and Vitamin D
- Protect your joints by avoiding undue stress such as high impact activity
- Exercise with range-of-motion, strength, and flexibility in mind

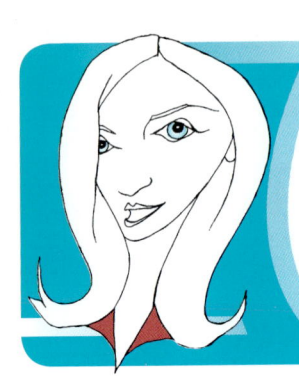

***CindySays***..."*Don't let osteoarthritis make you inactive. Respect the water's natural therapeutic benefits and allow it to be your exercise environment.*"

## Plunge Into a New Workout Arena

*The good news is you can still enjoy jogging, walking, toning, and stepping — all the variety of movement you want — if you simply do it in a pool. Water gives your body buoyancy and supports 90% of your bodyweight, thereby minimizing damaging stress to your joints.*

## There Are Cool Pool Toys That Add Resistance!

- Foam Weights
- Hand Paddles
- Jogging Belts
- Inflatable rubber mitts
- Fins and Cuffs

## Great Benefits of Water Exercise

- **Powerful plyometric movements** that would injure you on land remain powerful in the water but with minimal impact on your joints
- **You do not need to be able to swim** as flotation belts can be used for deep-water exercise and most activity is done in shallow water

- You can enjoy workouts indoor and outdoor depending on weather
- Children love the pool which makes it is a natural way for families to be active together
- Range of motion in the water is preserved and oftentimes increased due to buoyancy
- Progression of osteoarthritis is declines if activity is performed in water
- Water work can be either competitive (swim team sports) or non-competitive (group classes, freestyle), as you desire
- Helps control weight and conditions the heart and lungs

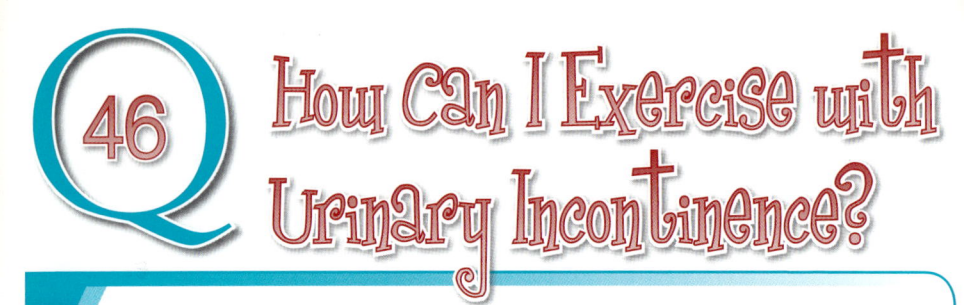

# Q46 How Can I Exercise with Urinary Incontinence?

**There are many causes for this common problem.** Pregnancy, childbirth, obesity, menopause, urinary tract infection, surgery, and pelvic injury can place physical stresses on the bladder and trigger ***Stress Urinary Incontinence (UI).*** The biggest myth is that it is a natural consequence of aging. It is true, however, that it is terribly aggravating and interferes with everyday activity.

## *The Best Prescription Is Exercise*

People with Stress UI are most likely to experience problems when they have a sudden increase in intra-abdominal pressure, which affects the bladder and bladder control. Quite often when someone coughs, laughs, sneezes, jumps, or lifts something heavy, it will cause urine leakage.

If life's events have taken a toll and there is muscle laxity, you must strengthen the muscles that hold the bladder in place so when everyday exertion occurs; these muscles are capable of handling the pressure.

## *Let's Talk Pelvic Fitness*

*Two main areas need attention. Here's how to identify the muscles that need strengthening*

- Try stopping the flow of urine mid-stream. If you can—you have identified one of the areas
- Imagine trying to stop passing gas. If you sense a pulling in the rectal area—you have identified the second area

*Remember what muscles you used to do the before-mentioned exercises.*

- Tighten these muscles for a count of ten and then release—these are known as Kegel Exercises
- Repeat this for five minutes, three times a day, making certain you do not tighten other muscles such as your stomach or legs
- Do not hold your breath as you do this
- Limit caffeine as it can make UI worse

**Be patient. It will take three to six weeks to feel a difference as with any muscle strengthening work.** But the rewards are great and those five minutes can be intermingled in your day without any fuss or preparation in doing so. In the meantime, you can still exercise. Using resistance machines and/or free weights along with non-impact cardiovascular machines, such as a stationary bike, can keep you fit while allowing you bathroom breaks when needed.

# 47 What Can I Do About Tennis Elbow?

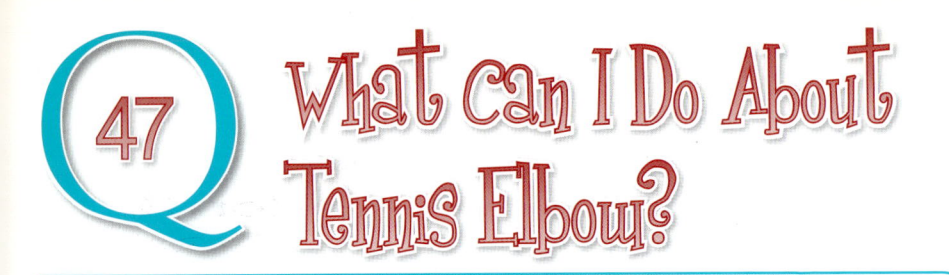

**This is an irritating affliction** is shared by many tennis enthusiasts. It is a condition that can sometimes cause people like you to hang up your racquet for good! It is a form of tendonitis.

## Symptoms of Tennis Elbow

- Pain on the outside portion of the elbow
- Pain increases when the tender area is pressed
- Pain when grasping, gripping or twisting objects
- Pain with activities that extend the wrist

## Keyword Here is PAIN!

- More painful in the evening making sleep difficult
- The elbow may be stiff in the morning
- Eventually even mild activity such as picking up a coffee cup, or turning a door knob is painful

Tennis like many other sports such as golf, baseball, racquetball, squash, and bowling is a *one-sided sport* (primarily using one side of the body). It is an activity comprised of *constant repetitive motion.* Consequently, it often uses and overuses your swinging arm until there are tiny tears in

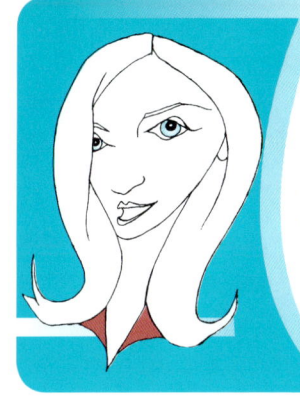

**CindySays**... *"Countless weekend athletes and/or "summer athletes" who intermittently take up demanding sports without proper conditioning, will suffer the consequences which can range from mild discomfort to chronic pain and serious injury. Expecting your body to perform painlessly under these conditions is unrealistic."*

the tendons of your forearm. Pain comes from *overusing* an area of the body, specifically, the elbow, which is unaccustomed to the continuous recurring movement.

## Prevention of Tennis Elbow

- Lift objects with *your palm facing your body*
- Strengthening exercises with hand weights—Begin with low weights and slowly progress to heavier weights
- Using light weights with *your elbow cocked and your palm down* repeatedly bend your wrist—Stop if you feel any pain
- Perform strength *work with resistance bands or tubing* to benefit the connective tissue of the joints
- Prior to playing tennis, *spend at least 10 minutes warming up* and follow it with a *mild stretch*
- Isometric exercises for the forearm and hand will improve grip control and minimize the effects of ball impact
- Hold a tennis ball in your palm—*Squeeze the ball firmly and hold for 3 seconds*-then relax—Repeat until your muscles fatigue

- Finger extension exercises will strengthen your hand—Place a thick rubber band around fingers and thumb near the base of fingers—*With palm facing the floor spread fingers apart as much as possible*—Hold 3 seconds- release—Repeat until hand fatigues
- Perform these exercises *3-4 times a week for 30-40 minutes*

## Treatment for Tennis Elbow

- Rest arm to allow the tendon to heal—Keep in mind it is an over-use injury
- Apply ice on affected area for 20 minutes to reduce swelling
- Anti-inflammatory medication, such as aspirin or ibuprofen may reduce discomfort
- If symptoms don't subside in two to four weeks, see a doctor or physical therapist

## Other Causes for Tennis Elbow

- Swinging late
- Not striking the ball in the center of the racquet strings
- Failing to use your lower body for power
- Using poor swing mechanics
- String tension
- Racquet weight, and grip size relevant to your size, ability and swing speed.

Finally, make an attempt to play year round so it becomes a ***"regular"*** activity. Playing only a few months a year barely gets the body acclimated to the demands that tennis places on muscles and joints. ***Tennis is a wonderful sport that most anyone can play for life*** if attention is paid to conditioning the body with sufficient strength and flexibility exercise.

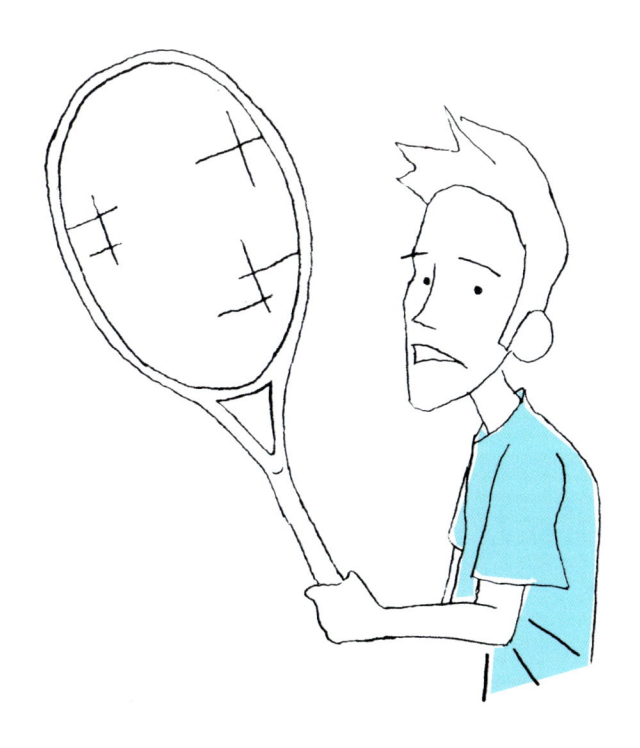

# Q48 Will Resistance Training Help Diabetics?

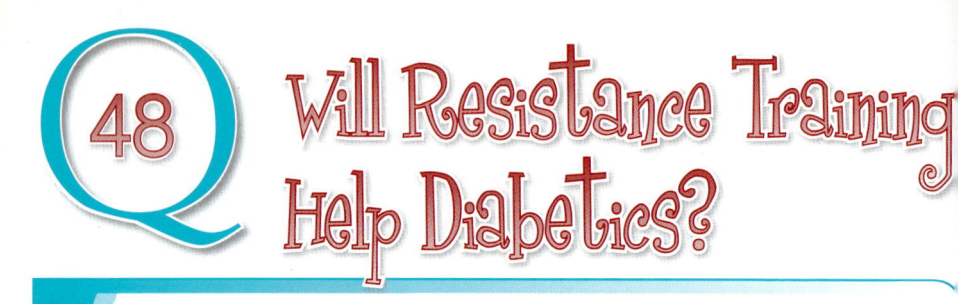

**Yes!** Anything you can perform safely that qualifies as physical activity is a positive move with regard to controlling your diabetes. Many approach fitness solely with a cardiovascular focus because for so many years it has be believed that weight loss could only be achieved by making our heart pump hard…ex. walking, running, swimming, stair-stepping or cycling. But progress is being made in convincing those who want to improve their physical condition that **weight training** is the key to many wonderful health benefits also.

## What Is Insulin Resistance?

The American Diabetes Association defines *insulin resistance* as the body's inability to respond to and use the insulin it produces. A diabetic who has insulin resistance has cells that are not responding to insulin appropriately therefore, the sugar in their blood cannot get into their cells. 1 in 4 people (without diabetes) has a genetic predisposition for insulin resistance. Whether or not the insulin resistance develops depends (in large part) on eating and exercise habits. Not being physically active is a huge reason why insulin resistance occurs. In addition, gaining weight/body fat (especially around the middle) is a common trigger.

Before starting any new physical activity, always check with your doctor to ensure that it is safe. Some diabetes related conditions, such as eye or kidney damage may override the benefits.

## *How Does Weight Training Reduce Insulin Resistance?*

- Improves insulin sensitivity
- Increases muscle mass
- Reduces fat
- Trims Visceral fat which is linked to insulin resistance This type of exercise also trims visceral fat—fat that surrounds the organs, which is linked to insulin resistance

## *Other Benefits*

- Increases strength and endurance
- Increases bone density
- Decreases osteoarthritic symptoms
- Increases mobility
- Positively affects hypertension and lipid profiles

This is good news for diabetics who may be unable to perform cardiovascular exercise due to advancing age, obesity, existing joint problems or nerve damage to their feet.

So in addition to your swimming and miles on the treadmill, go ahead and pump it up! Regular physical activity (both aerobics and strength training) increase your cells' sensitivity to insulin.

## *What Does It Take?*

- Aim for 20-60 minutes of aerobic activity, *three to five days a week*
- 30 minutes of strength training *(with free weights, machines, resistance bands, or your own body's resistance)* two to three times a week
- Consistent physical activity will bring about a 10 % reduction in weight which will also *reduce insulin resistance*

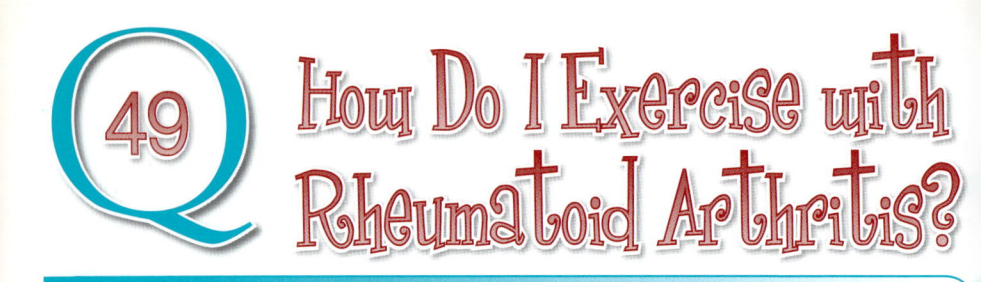

# Q49 How Do I Exercise with Rheumatoid Arthritis?

**Autoimmune disorders** such as the many types of arthritis and lupus affect your supporting structures (muscles—tendons—ligaments) and cause joint pain, stiffness, swelling, and inflammation. Because people affected by these require a good deal of rest, many assume they should not exercise. However, getting adequate amounts of activity is extremely important in terms of pain and fatigue management and progression of the disorder. Inactivity, in fact, may increase the problems associated with arthritis and lupus.

## Managing Arthritis Is the Key

Learning to incorporate the right amount of movement, will allow you to have a more active lifestyle and keep you in control of the disease. The trick is to find a balance of rest and exercise.

## Your Movement Should Incorporate Three Types of Exercise

Cardio respiratory (heart and lung) conditioning
- *Swim-Walk-Cycle-Treadmills-Ellipticals-Rowers*

Strengthening exercises or muscle endurance
- *Light Training-Resistance Machines-Bands-Free Weights-Yoga*

Flexibility work to preserve full range of motion in joints
- *Stretching-Tai Chi-Yoga-Water Movement*

## Benefits of Exercise

1. Moderate activity has emotional benefits-it not only reduces pain and other physical related symptoms but also improves mood as pain can cause depression.
2. Exercise helps you manage your weight alleviating undue stress on joints
3. Energy increases in active people
4. The right amount of activity will reduce arthritis and lupus flare-ups
5. Reduces joint pain and inflammation and improve overall sense of well-being

## Precautions

1. If you have been inactive see your health care professional for assistance in prescribing the proper amount of exercise
2. Begin slowly and progress gradually
3. Mild to moderate intensities are the rule of thumb
4. Exercise that causes pain lasting for more than an hour is too intense

# Q50 Why Do My Bendable Parts Crack and Pop?

**Parts such as the knees, neck, ankles, knuckles and back** are known to make all sorts of noises during movement and can be quite disturbing. Some of these sounds can be serious but most are not indicative of any real underlying problem. Usually the popping is attributable to one of three commonly accepted explanations.

## Why We Snap Crackle and Pop

- *Escaping gases:* Synovial fluid in joints acts as a lubricant: This fluid contains oxygen, nitrogen, and carbon dioxide. When you bend, stretch or activate the joint, the joint capsule stretches and forms gas bubbles that when released create these noises.

- *Movement of joints, tendons and ligaments:* When a joint moves, the tendon's position changes and moves slightly out of place. A snapping sound is heard as the tendon returns to its original position. In addition, the ligaments may tighten as joints move. This commonly occurs in knees or ankles, and can make loud cracking sounds.

- *Rough surfaces:* Arthritic joints make sounds caused by the loss of smooth cartilage and the roughness of the joint surface.

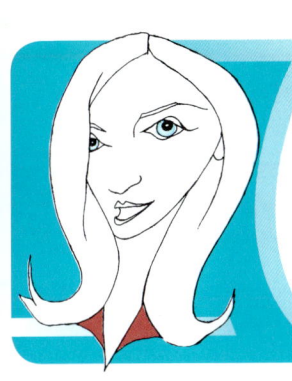

***CindySays***... "*Most popping and cracking occurs after a period of rest and inactivity, so let that be a lesson to keep the body moving.*"

## *Bark Usually Worse Than the Bite*

But, don't rely on a specific sound to diagnosis the severity. See an orthopedic doctor if in addition to popping, you have:

- Pain
- Swelling
- Limitations of normal movement

They will evaluate the integrity of the joint in question and make the appropriate call. If there is no pain or swelling of the joint during or after activity, you probably have little reason for concern. Maintaining muscular strength and flexibility around the knees along with conditioning with weights may be helpful to further improve leg strength and automatically decrease the amount of stress on the knees. This will allow for smoother and more reliable movement of the joint.

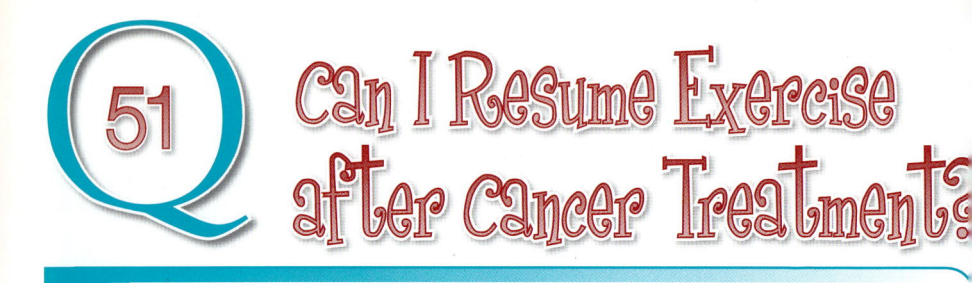

## Q51 Can I Resume Exercise after Cancer Treatment?

**Some people are able to remain active throughout treatment,** but many are not. If you have been inactive for an extended period of time, you probably are eager to resume normal activities. Once you have finished treatment, your physician will give you the green light with regard to adding regular physical activity back in. The amount of time you were sedentary, however, will determine how quickly this should be done. The longer you were inactive, the more gradual the process should be. Ease back into activity, in terms of quantity and intensity of exercise, to allow your body the necessary time to adjust, which, in turn, will restore your energy and sense of well-being.

### Added Benefits of Exercise

- Speeds recovery
- Builds strength and endurance
- Reduces anxiety and feelings of depression
- Facilitates restful sleep
- Improves self-esteem and lightens mood
- Builds energy
- Strengthens immune system

## Listen to Your Body

Your focus should be on taking small steps. The recommendation of 30 minutes of exercise five or more days a week is just that—a recommendation. If this amount of activity is causing unusual fatigue or pain, adjust the intensity or frequency down until your energy level catches up with your desire to be stronger. *Do what you can, even if it is a 5 or 10-minute walk* and be proud of that. Following your treatments, each day will be an improvement.

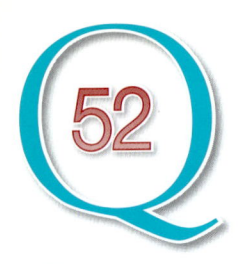

# 52. How Can I Ease the Pain in my Side When I Run?

Side stitches just below the rib cage are annoyingly common and have been the subject of many studies. *Exercise Related Transient Abdominal Pain or ETAP* is believed to be the result when ligaments are stretched that run from the diaphragm to other organs, particularly the liver and stomach.

## Causes of Side Stitches

**Excessive jolting motion from activities** involving up and down movement such as running, jumping or horseback riding while breathing causes ligaments to stretch

**Studies show most people exhale** as their left foot strikes the ground. These people are less affected by ETAP than those who exhale when their right foot strikes the ground

*Exhaling when the right foot strikes the ground generates greater trauma to the liver which is positioned just below the rib cage on the right side of the body. Just as the liver is dropping down, the exhalation causes the diaphragm to raise up which brings about spasms and ETAP.*

## Prevention of ETAP

- Avoid eating one to two hours prior to your workout
- Start slow and progress gradually
- Take consistent deep breaths
- Make sure you are well hydrated

## Try These Methods

- Slow your pace or walk longer to achieve a better warm up
- Reach your right arm up and lean to the left for a good stretch
- Massage in the area of the muscle spasm
- Stop moving—exhale as you place your hand on right side of belly and lift up
- Bend forward to stretch the diaphragm
- Always consult a physician if pain persists

# 53 How Do I Exercise Safely in the Heat?

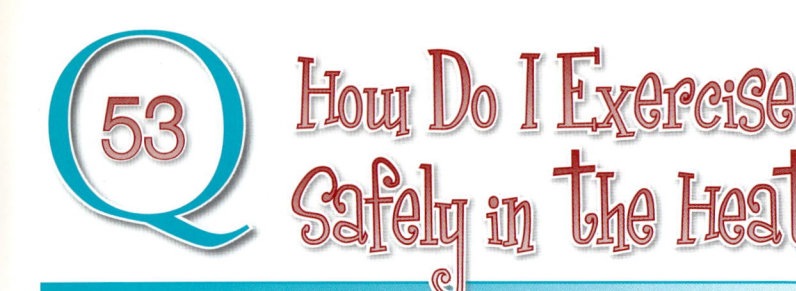

**Exercising outside in warm weather offers** more than fitness. It combines scenic nature and a variety of terrains to make your workout interesting and ever-changing.

However, heat and humidity must be taken into account as it can have a major effect on your health and safety. Your body needs time to adjust to the outdoor temperature and humidity levels. *"Getting used to"* or acclimated to the uncontrolled temperatures should be done gradually and progressively. It takes most people seven to ten days of repeated exposure to heat for the body to safely acclimate to the change in the environment.

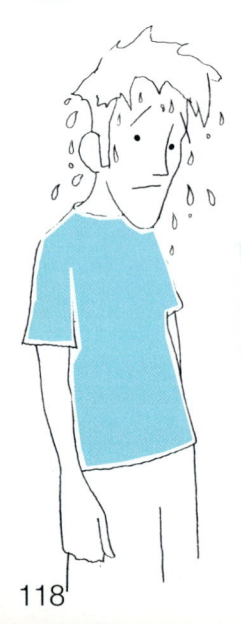

Drinking plenty of water prior to your outdoor activities is essential and it is just as important to continue drinking 6 to 8 ounces of water every 15 to 20 minutes. This will make a tremendous difference in your heart's ability to adapt to the heat and stress.

## Consider What Stresses Your Body When Exercising Outside

1. Air temperature
2. Humidity level
3. Hydration level
4. Length and intensity of workout

*A 90 degree day with 80% humidity is equal to 113 degrees to your body!*

## Symptoms of Heat Illness

- Dizziness
- Headache
- Fatigue
- Chills
- Tachycardia
- Diarrhea
- Nausea
- Leg Cramps
- Feeling as if something is NOT RIGHT

**IMPORTANT**-*If any one of these is present, stop the workout, remove yourself from the heat and drink water!*

**It is difficult to say *how hot is too hot.*** It is different for everyone. Use caution—move your fitness workouts to the beautiful outdoors with forethought and preparation. Increase the amount of time outdoors gradually in order to safely increase your body's heat tolerance.

# 54 What Are Good Exercises For People With MS?

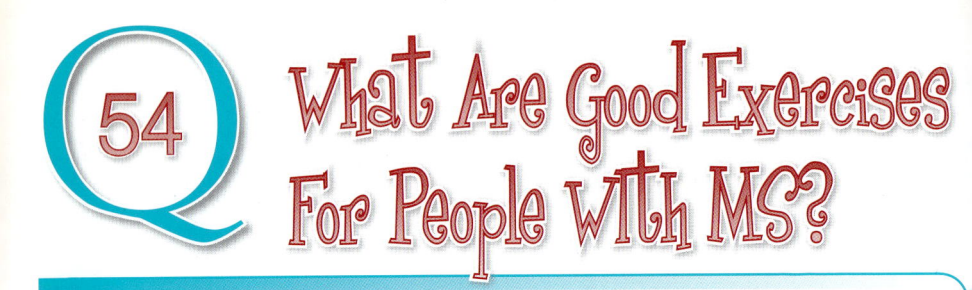

**Multiple sclerosis or MS is a *chronic, unpredictable neurological disease that affects the central nervous system.*** While most people with MS do not become severely disabled, they do have challenges they must be attentive to. There is joint stiffness, pain, fatigue and weakness that translate into functional mobility deficits.

**The symptoms and severity differ** from one person to the next so what may be a problem for some may not be for another. The unique way MS affects each individual on any given day makes it a bad idea to offer cookie cutter solutions.

## *Paying Attention to the Body*

Working out too intensely causes those with MS to overheat which can make symptoms worse. Very cold weather can do the same. Most people with MS should be mindful of their body temperature as it plays an important role in how they feel day to day. Not everyone with MS is affected by extreme temperatures. But for some, even a difference of one-quarter to one-half of a degree can cause problems. Those who are heat sensitive or basically have a malfunctioning internal thermostat can have muscle spasms, pain, weakness and slurred speech if they become too hot or too cold.

*What can a heat-sensitive person do who wants to exercise but does not want to suffer the consequences of increased body temperature?*

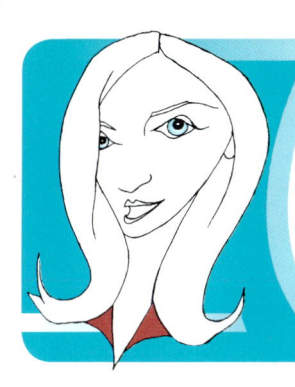

**CindySays...** *"Activities such as gentle yoga, light intensity strength-training, and aquatics are ideal for those living actively with Multiple Sclerosis. Staying active with appropriate activity will offer valuable functional benefits and a feeling of well-being."*

## Try to Avoid

- Hot environments including hot tubs and showers, hot outdoor temperatures and direct sunlight
- Prolonged or intense activity
- Hot drinks or foods
- Heavy or constrictive clothing

## Suggestions if You Can't Avoid Extreme Temperatures

- Wear light layers of clothing and shed layers as your body temperature increases
- Exercise in an air-conditioned environment
- Drink approximately 8 oz. of water 8 times a day
- Wear properly fitted footwear that allows your feet to breathe
- Eat light meals often as heavy meals will increase body temperature
- Find a variety of exercise that is light to moderate in intensity
- Doing workouts in a pool (ideally 80 to 84 degrees) is optimum for those with MS
- Alternate periods of exercise with equal periods of rest
- Wear special clothes that cool the body for more rigorous workouts

# Q55 I Have Varicose Veins—Should I Exercise?

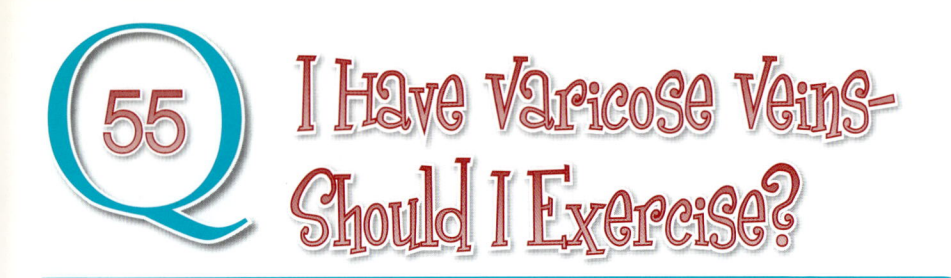

Actually quite common—40% of women and 25% of men have significant vein circulation problems, clinically known as *chronic venous insufficiency,* by the time they reach the age of 40, and this incidence increases with age.

## Not Simply a Result of Aging

- Varicose veins are lumpy, winding, and sometimes twisted vessels just below the surface of the skin and occur when valves between the deep and superficial veins of the leg no longer function properly
- Symptoms include swelling, muscle cramps, aching, throbbing, burning, itching, and heaviness in the legs
- There are multiple causes of varicose veins, including heredity, lifestyle, over-weight and obesity, age, hormones, leg trauma, pregnancy, birth control, and hormonal replacement therapy
- They occur quite often in young women following pregnancy
- Varicose veins should not to be confused with spider veins, which look like spider legs and are principally cosmetic. Spider veins rarely lead to complications associated with varicose veins
- Varicose veins are frequently a medical risk because they can cause phlebitis, blood clots, varicosity hemorrhaging, stasis dermatitis, and venous ulcers

## Exercise Is a Good Thing

- **Maintaining a healthy body weight** and getting adequate exercise are two of the most beneficial things you can do for yourself in terms of lessening the progression of varicose veins
- **While long periods of standing or sitting is detrimental,** moving the legs and staying active is what will alleviate symptoms and improve venous circulation to the normal deep vein systems in the thigh and calf muscles
- **Getting off your feet** is a valid recommendation—at the end of the day and when at rest—but movement of the legs is necessary
- **Properly warming up and cooling down is vital;** otherwise symptoms might be aggravated
- **Choose an activity that is tolerable,** such as walking, jogging, strength training, cycling, swimming, water walking, yoga, dancing, or a sport
- **If a typical day requires sitting at a desk** or standing for extended time, take frequent breaks to move your legs, especially the calf muscles
- **If you must remain seated,** elevate your legs as much as possible, and do heel raises—*point and flex your toes throughout the day*

## Dramatically Simplified Treatment

- **There are several minimally invasive procedures** that successfully treat the pain and symptoms of varicosities
- **EVLT** or endovenous laser therapy is non-surgical and uses laser heat to obliterate the affected vein
- **Sclerotherapy** is another treatment process using chemicals injected into small to medium-sized veins
- **Radio-frequency closure** uses radio energy as a heat source to destroy the vein

All of these treatments replace previous, traditional vein surgeries, and no longer require hospital stays or extensive recovery periods. Eliminating the persistent pain and other unpleasant symptoms associated with varicosities is certainly a step in the right direction toward a healthy and more active life.

## Q56 How Do I Avoid the Germs in the Gym?

**A typical workout facility can be a breeding ground for germs** that are as strong as the biceps and triceps they live on. In fact, germs love the gym—actually they love the moisture present in the shower stalls, pools, steam rooms, and just plain old sweat. It can make you wonder if you are doing more damage than good going to a crowded gym.

**The moisture is the incubator** for the germs left behind by facility users. They grow in this warm environment and are then passed along when you come in contact with these breeding grounds. Don't panic yet—there is only a small possibility these germs will become a health hazard especially if regular cleaning and sanitization is performed.

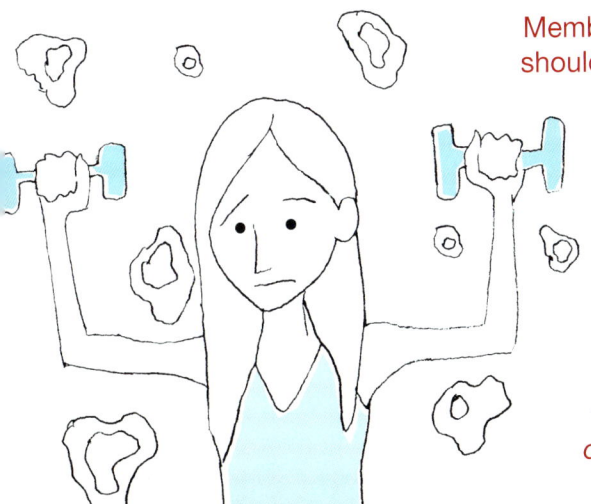

**Members at workout centers should be involved** by asking that the environment they train in be as germ free as possible. This job, however, cannot be done by the gym staff alone. It requires mutual cooperation by those working for the gym as well as those *working out in* the gym.

## SHARE THE RESPONSIBILITY
### Exercise Facility Expectations

- **Keep workout areas well ventilated** to prevent stale air from being continually recycled
- **Clean the entire facility regularly** with a disinfectant solution
- **Make spray disinfectants or wipes readily available** to members to ensure equipment is continually cleaned
- **Adhere to hot tub, whirlpool and swimming pools inspections** to make certain that proper levels of germ-fighting chlorine and bromine are maintained
- **Make certain locker rooms,** bathrooms, saunas and steam rooms are similarly cleaned and inspected
- **Encourage anyone** (staff or members) to stay away from the gym when they are sick
- **Supply clean towels** and make it mandatory for members to wipe off their equipment when leaving it for the next member
- **Identify the areas of most concern and clean them more often**—like stair-climber and bicycle grips, doorknobs, weights and water fountain handles

Most workout facilities are aware of what it takes to maintain a sanitary gym environment and are diligent about it. But, even impeccable cleaning regimens can miss determined germs. This is where the members must take some responsibility in this effort.

### Member Expectations

- **Always bring two different looking towels** (so you can keep them separate) from home—one to wipe the sweat from your body and one to wipe your equipment down once you've finished using it

- **Cover any scrapes or abrasions with a band-aid** before going to the gym
- **Once your workout begins never touch your face**—nose, eyes, mouth—until you're workout is completed and you have washed your hands thoroughly
- **Use disinfectant supplied by the gym** to spray your equipment—if it is not supplied—ask for it or bring your own
- **Wear shower slippers or flip flops** on pool decks, showers, saunas and steam-rooms
- **Bring a clean towel from home** to sit on if you use the steam room or sauna—flu season may not be the optimum time to use either of these rooms
- **If you are not feeling well stay away from the gym.** If you have cold symptoms (from the chin up) take a week off and (from the chin down) take two weeks off
- **Carry a gym bag that is washable and wash it often.** Take sweaty towels and clothing out of the bag and wash after each workout
- **Wash your hands thoroughly before and after your workout**
- **Carry an alcohol based hand sanitizer to use if you feel the need**

**With all that in mind, it may not seem worth it.** But, if you are otherwise healthy, it IS worth going. Maintaining your fitness level is the way you stimulate your immune system. Regular workouts are your greatest ally in this germ warfare.

**Go to the gym prepared to practice good gym etiquette.** It is up to you and the staff to share the responsibility so that you and others can stay healthy and strong all year long.

# Q57 Should I Work Out When I Am Sick?

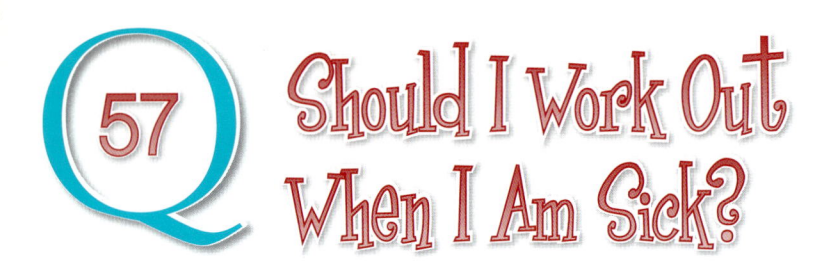

**Most sports medicine experts agree** the answer lies in the location of your symptoms.

## Discomfort Above the Neck

- **It is safe to engage in mild to moderate intensity activity** if your symptoms include head congestion, sneezing, scratchy throat, or headache or in general, *discomfort above the neck.*

## Symptoms Below the Neck

- **On the other hand,** if you have a fever, chest congestion, coughing, nausea, vomiting, or diarrhea, or *symptoms generated below the neck,* you should restrict exercise until these symptoms subside. If you are experiencing any of these, you may have a viral or bacterial infection, which is much more severe and requires rest.

## Listen to Your Body

- **Your body will usually tell you if it is up for exercise.** Forcing exercise on a body that is under the weather will typically come back to haunt you by making the condition worse. Remember that a recuperating body is getting a workout, whether or not you are actively participating.

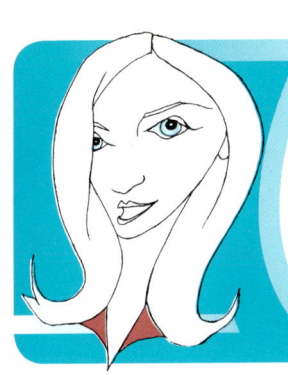

*CindySays*..."No question that adequate hydration is critical if you are not feeling 100% so make an extra effort to drink plenty of water."

## Return to Activity Slowly

- It is a good idea to resume your training at 50% of your usual exercise intensity. If after 15 to 20 minutes you are still feeling good, gradually increase intensity to 85 to 90%. *Important—if you feel worse after your initial warm up, throw in the towel and wait for another day.*

## Chapter 5

# FITNESS GADGETS AND THE MAGIC BULLET

**The good, the bad and the ridiculous** are advertised and touted as the missing link between you and that fabulous body of your dreams. The busier we are, the more we tend to seek out a better or more efficient way to live our lives. We seek shortcuts in business, travel, food preparation, relationships, and so why not in our pursuit of health?

**Sounds like a good idea** — in fact, it's a grand idea if we can purchase one tool or piece of equipment that will instantly make us feel better, look better and live longer. Unfortunately, this tool has never been invented. If we agree there is no magic bullet—then we must assess products individually and evaluate their claims in terms of sound fitness practice and safety.

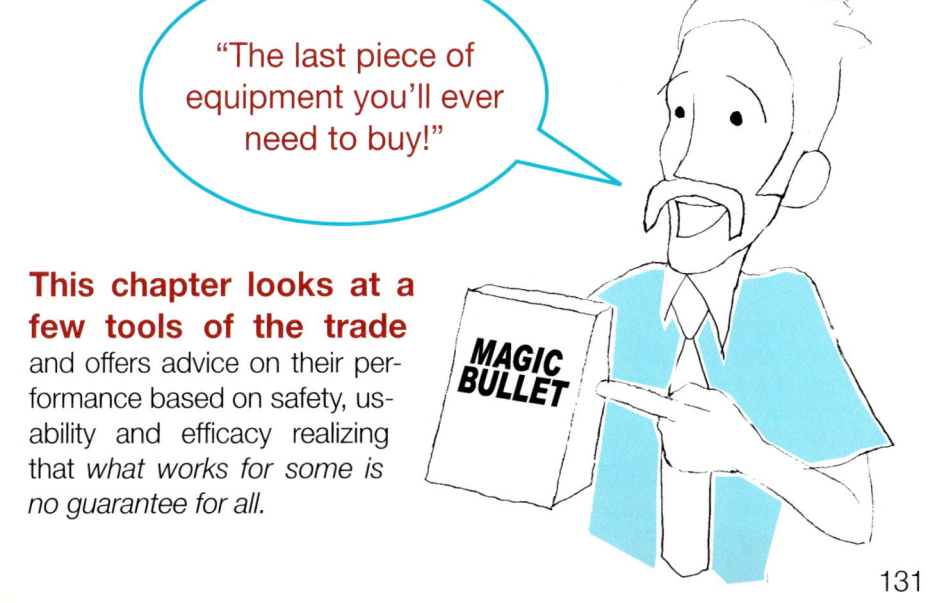

"The last piece of equipment you'll ever need to buy!"

**This chapter looks at a few tools of the trade** and offers advice on their performance based on safety, usability and efficacy realizing that *what works for some is no guarantee for all.*

# Q58 Do Ab Exercisers Really Work?

The abdominals connect your shoulders to your hips. In order to move with strength, balance, and grace, you must condition the abdominals. Some abdominal equipment has merit, **but beware— equipment that requires no physical effort from you other than swiping a credit card is worthless.**

- **Equipment that claims to do the work for you** such as electronic abdominal exercise belts which send electrical impulses to the body are a waste of your money and time. Studies show they are ineffective and can even be painful.

- **Some abdominal exercisers** successfully position or cradle the user. For those unsure about proper technique, these may be helpful.

- **A large exercise ball** (average size-55cm) is a good choice to facilitate quality abdominal and back training. It offers cushioned support while it demands the user to engage the stabilizer muscles of the core. While the crunches and extensions are more difficult to perform, they are also more targeted and therefore give you better results. The ball is excellent for stretching these muscles as well.

- **People generally ignore their abs completely** or over train them to a fault. Enviable abs and healthy backs are bestowed upon those who do 2 to 3 high quality sets of 15 reps rather than those who do hundreds.

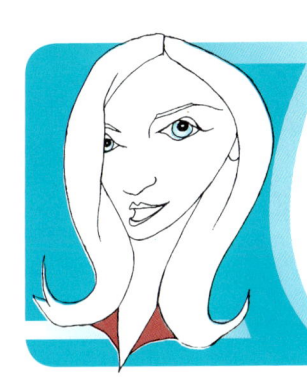

**CindySays**..."*Having commercial quality abs—six-pack abs—is more about good nutrition (70% responsible) than it is about reps. Even rock hard abs are quite good at hiding beneath excess layers of fat.*"

## CRUNCH INSTRUCTIONS

For a safe and effective abdominal crunch, lie on your back (with or without the ball) with knees bent and feet flat on floor. Place your fingers behind ears or across chest. Exhale as you raise your shoulders (imagine peeling one vertebrae at a time from the floor) until you feel resistance and contraction in your abdominal area. Inhale as you slowly lower your shoulders and head back to starting position. Perform 3 sets of 15 crunches with 15 second rests between sets.

# Q59 Who or What is a Bosu Trainer?

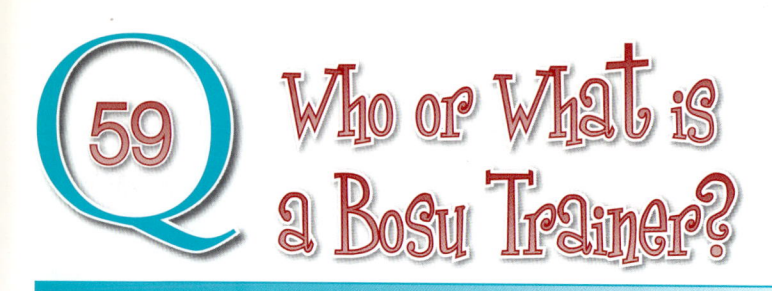

**The Bosu—stands for BOth Sides Up**—Ball or Trainer looks like a large ball that has been cut in half. It is a cross-training tool that works on stability, balance, and strength. Training is done from either side. Approximately 25 inches in diameter, one side is flat and the other is rounded or dome-shaped. It challenges the user to maintain their center of gravity because it is unstable and wobbly.

## *Best Aspects of the Bosu Ball*

- Versatility-Used for strength and core training, sports conditioning and agility
- Balance-Can target muscles that help stabilize the body
- Body Awareness-Develops a keen sense of body positioning during movement

## *Worst Aspects of the Bosu Ball*

- Often overused by fitness trainers who build entire training sessions around Bosu
- Limited with regard to overall fitness
- Though sometimes used in rehabilitative setting, it is not for everyone

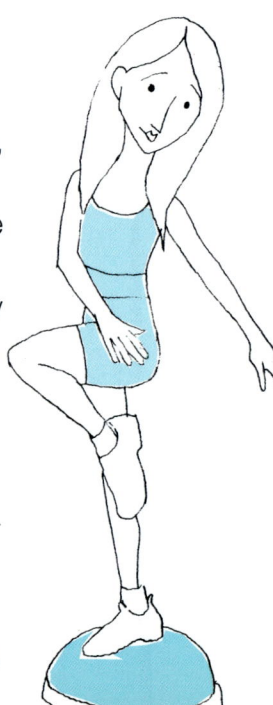

# 60 Why Buy Resistance Bands if I Have Weights?

Because each work your muscles and joints in a slightly different way. Bands and tubing offer **variable resistance** and free weights offer **constant resistance.** Neither one is better but each one can do something the other one cannot.

- Variable resistance-The amount of resistance an exercise tube or band exerts on a muscle increases as it is stretched. It may start out at five pounds of resistance but as you pull or stretch it—the resistance may increase to eight pounds. The longer you make it—the more force it puts on the muscle.
- Constant resistance -The amount of resistance a ten pound dumbbell (free weight) puts on a muscle will continue to be ten pounds throughout the full range of motion of an exercise.

## *Both Are Beneficial*

Free weights like dumbbells stimulate more muscles to work simply to maintain proper form during the movement. They are also available in many more weight increments which is better for those who strength-train with heavier weight. *Free weights therefore are going to be more beneficial if you want to build muscle strength.*

Resistance tubes and bands are ideal for anyone new at strength training because the variable resistance quality challenges the exerciser at their current level of strength. Often, you will see bands used in a reha-

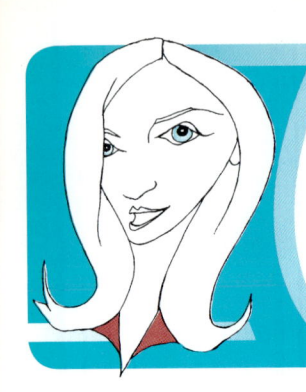

> **CindySays**... "Exercise bands and tubes are inexpensive, extremely lightweight and compact—a great tool to carry with you for workouts on the run."

bilitative setting because they encourage joint stability. The bands and tubes also have the advantage of offering resistance in multiple directions, which is useful in sports specific training as they can add resistance to a simulated sport movement. *Bands and tubes are going to be beneficial with beginners, in therapeutic use, and sports training.*

Incorporating both weights and bands into your strength training regimen can build strong bones, durable joints and prevent boredom from doing the same old thing over and over again.

# Q61 What Is a Rebounder?

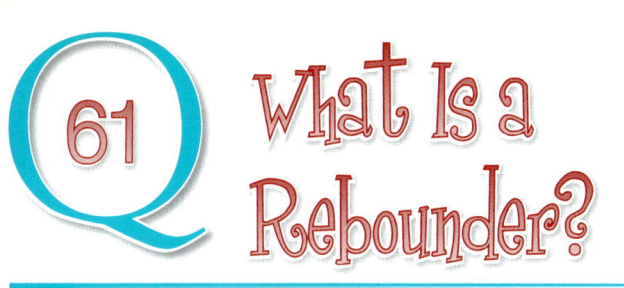

**The apparatus known as the Rebounder is an updated version of the mini-trampoline** now finding its way into homes and fitness centers. It can be quite intense and athletic oriented. Because it is a relatively small working surface—average of 28 inches—the Rebounder requires the exerciser to maintain balance and core stability while jumping up and down. However, it usually comes with a stability bar attachment to hold on to during which lessens the risk of falling or bounding off.

## Considerations before Purchasing on the Rebound

- **Rebounding is cardiovascular** so it can condition your heart and lungs.

- **It is a great weight bearing (bone building) choice.** Your bones feel the effects of three times your weight on each landing with less impact on your joints than running.

- **Athletic people are more inclined to enjoy this form of exercise** because they have a well-developed sense of balance, coordination, rhythm, timing, and dexterity.

- **Less athletically gifted people may be somewhat intimidated** by the demands of the rebounding movement as it may evoke an out of control feeling.

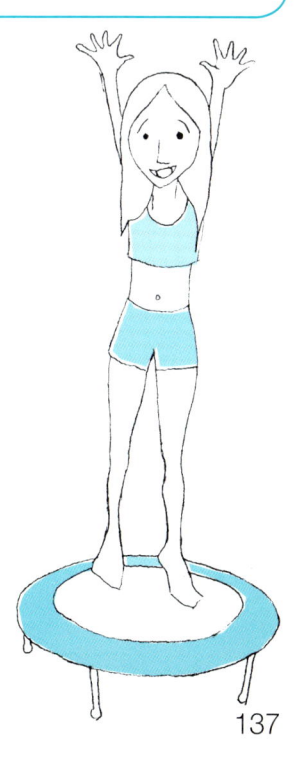

- While the landing surface is unstable, it is resilient and therefore, easy on the joints—most of the shock—*close to 90%*—is absorbed by the apparatus.
- Those with weak ankles or knee problems may have difficulty on this unstable surface and risk rolling an ankle or twisting a knee if landings are off-center.

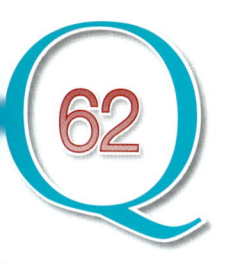

## Q62 Should I Join the Dance Dance Revolution?

**If you like to dance and want to get fit** while having fun…then by all means get involved in the revolution. **Dance Dance Revolution or DDR** is one of the most effective weapons against childhood obesity. Historically, young people who are overweight, shy away from traditional sports and exercise. DDR has put a new spin on exercise by adding hip music (chosen by player) to the video game concept. Players move their feet on a special mat as directed by arrows that scroll on a TV monitor. Players must step on the same symbols on the mat at just the right time to score well.

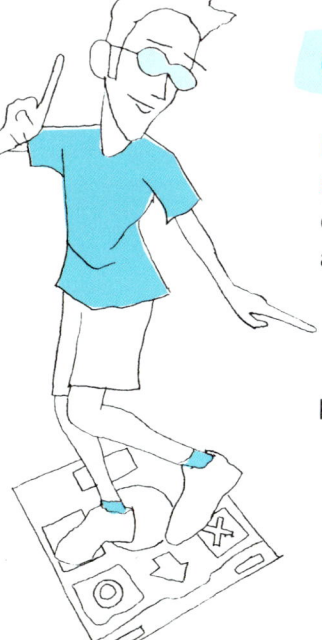

### Good News!!

**DDR is now finding its way into public school systems** and while it does not replace physical education and health classes it is one more activity option on the curriculum menu. *It is not just for kids*—adults who are bored with treadmills, ellipticals and rowing machines might find DDR just the help they need to pull them from the dreaded exercise rut.

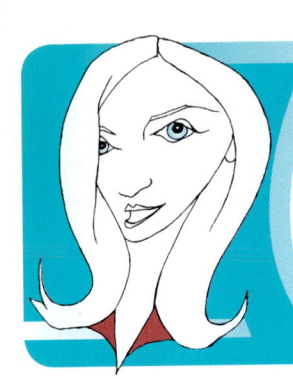

*CindySays...* "Whether you're young or old get your groove on and join the revolution."

## Benefits of DDR

- **Cardiovascular**—Players progressively challenge their heart and lungs
- **Burns Calories**—Can be an enjoyable way to achieve a healthy body weight
- **Lower Body Conditioning**—Hips and legs get a great workout
- **Agility**—Trains players reaction time and quickness

# Q63 Are Cardiovascular Machines Worth Buying?

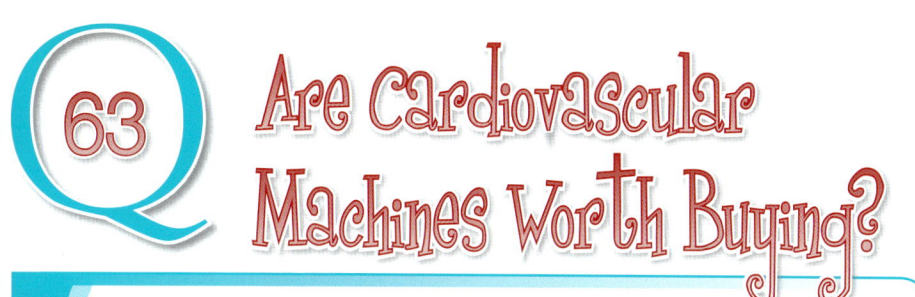

**Of course they are if you use them.** Having any kind of equipment in your home seems like a terrific idea. After all, we lead busy lives in hectic worlds. Owning a cardio machine, such as a treadmill, elliptical, rower, stair-stepper or stationary bike can theoretically be a shortcut for us. However, many find they rarely use them in the home after the first six months of the purchase. They become dust catchers, clothes hangers and ultimately a bad buy. Still, there are some who will use the equipment and for these people, putting together a home gym is an excellent use of space.

If you have never owned equipment or worked out in your home, please consider this advice prior to making that financial commitment for one or more cardio machines.

## Test Drive the Idea of Home Equipment

- Test the waters to determine if home exercise works for you
- Try a less expensive model the first time
- Choose a simple cardio machine without the bells and whistles
- Equipment with "extras" drive the price up but don't guarantee superior results

There are hundreds of treadmills for instance offering lots of bells and whistles, but more often than not, those bells and whistles very seldom get rung or tooted. Most regular treadmill walkers come to value simpler things like durability, ample striding area that is cushioned for impact, automatic power shut-off in case of a slip or fall, and ease of programming. This is true for any cardio machine.

## *Cardio Equipment Suggestions*

- Used equipment is a great place to start—and it is usually like new as the sellers are selling it because they never used it
- Try the equipment out before you buy—take your running shoes to the store and actually go for a walk or run
- Once you determine you consistently exercise in the home—gradually add other equipment such as free weights, resistance bands and weight bench

Buying fitness equipment is a decision that requires some comparison research as well as some actual personal testing. A little legwork will go a long way in helping you to make a wise treadmill choice and will be worth it over the long haul.

# 64 How Can a Heart Rate Monitor Help Me?

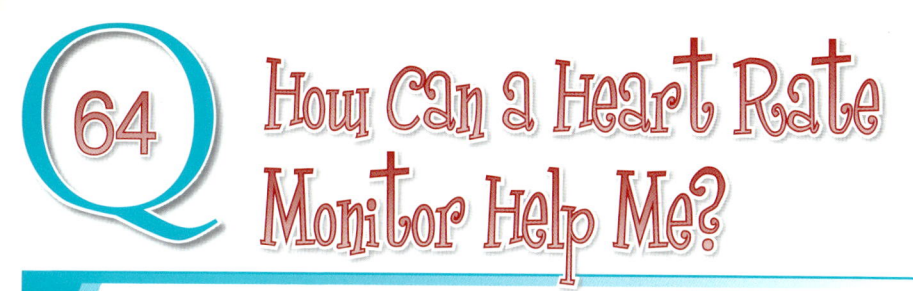

**You can make dramatic improvements in your health** with regular exercise. Just 30 to 60 minutes most days of the week will improve cardiovascular health, decrease blood pressure, raise good cholesterol, lower bad cholesterol, facilitate weight loss, and prevent many forms of chronic disease. However, the intensity level of this activity is important. A heart rate monitor can ensure you are working within your target heart rate range—one that is challenging enough but at the same time safe.

## Heart Rate Monitors vs. Taking Own Pulse

Yes, you can take your pulse by placing two fingers on your wrist. Fitness classes teach you to do this and it is a good ritual to get into. But, if you believe in wearing supportive shoes and breathable clothing during physical activity, you should also value a tool that provides you with an accurate heart rate.

- Heart rate monitors don't need be elaborate—bells and whistles are rarely used
- Digital heart rate monitors are nice as they won't pick up heart rates nearby
- Heart rate monitors help prevent overtraining and decrease injury risk

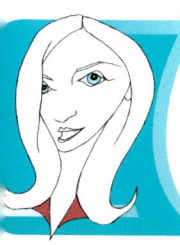

*CindySays…"Considering the myriad of fitness tools on the market to choose from—a heart rate monitor is a smart investment that can assist you in optimal cardiovascular training."*

# Q65 What Is a Power Plate and Does It Work?

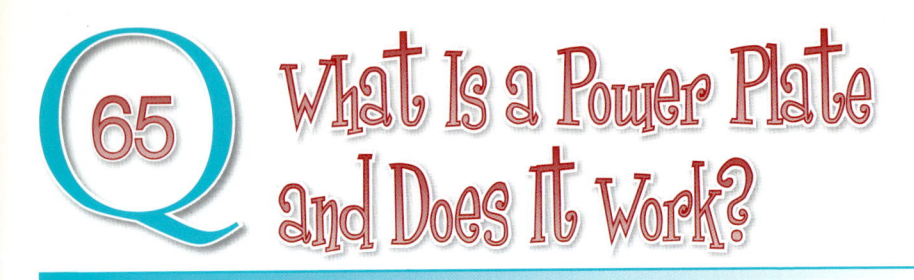

**This power plate is advertised for seasoned athletes** as well as older adults. It claims to vibrate the body into shape by initiating the stretch reflex. Just fifteen minutes three days a week will theoretically take your entire body to a new level of fitness. The vibrations are said to cause the body to transmit waves of energy that activate muscles and cause contractions. It is a pricey gadget with little in the way of science to support its claims.

## Buyer Beware

Standing on a machine that shakes you may wake you up and make you feel like you are active but the truth is unless you exert physical energy you will not burn calories or strengthen muscles.

## Here's the Problem

Instructions give the buyer exercises to do while on the power plate. Hmmm—wouldn't I just be as well off doing these without a shaky floor beneath me? Oh, it may challenge your balance a little and make each of the prescribed exercises slightly more difficult but is that worth the high price tag? You be the judge—as for me, I'll keep my money and perform the exercise on a floor, bosu ball or if I am really daring, on a mechanical bull.

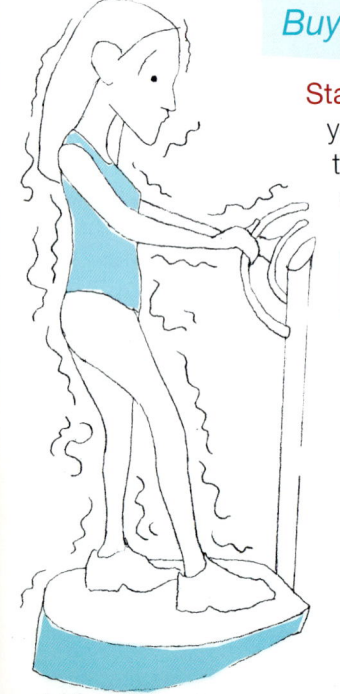

# Q66 What Home Equipment Should I Invest In?

Any equipment you use on a regular basis is valuable and worth the investment. Likewise, any equipment, regardless of its price or potential, is worthless if it goes unused. Look in any classified ad section of a newspaper and you will see how many barely used pieces of good equipment are for sale at bargain basement prices.

**If you have never exercised in your home,** think twice about buying costly equipment in the beginning. Instead, purchase inexpensive tools first such as dumbbells or an exercise ball to see if you establish a regular in-home training habit. If you do, then investing in quality equipment is a great idea.

**If you work out at a gym,** you will benefit from the equipment listed below for occasional in-home training. There will always be times when you cannot get to the fitness center. Spending 30 minutes on basic exercises with free weights will help keep your exercise regimen in tact.

## *Home Workout Basics*

- Dumbbells and Resistance Bands
- Workout bench
- Exercise ball
- Stretching mat
- Heart Rate Monitor
- Pedometer
- Optional-Cardiovascular Equipment

## Chapter 6
# THE SKINNY ON EATING FOR HEALTH

**Is it any wonder there is growing confusion** considering the many food choices and ever-changing diets? Low-fat, no-fat, low-carb, high protein, sugar-free, supplementation, eating disorders, fast foods, slow-cooked are just a few of the half-baked ideas and terminology found in our hectic world. Dialogues change monthly in terms of what is good for us and what is bad for us. Last month's good foods are now bad foods.

**Add to this the invisible line of demarcation** between nutrition and fitness. Nutrition experts rarely mention fitness and vice-versa. Even worse, however, is the unfortunate scenario of the fitness expert professing to be an expert in dietary needs and the nutritional expert failing to understand the dietary needs of extremely active people.

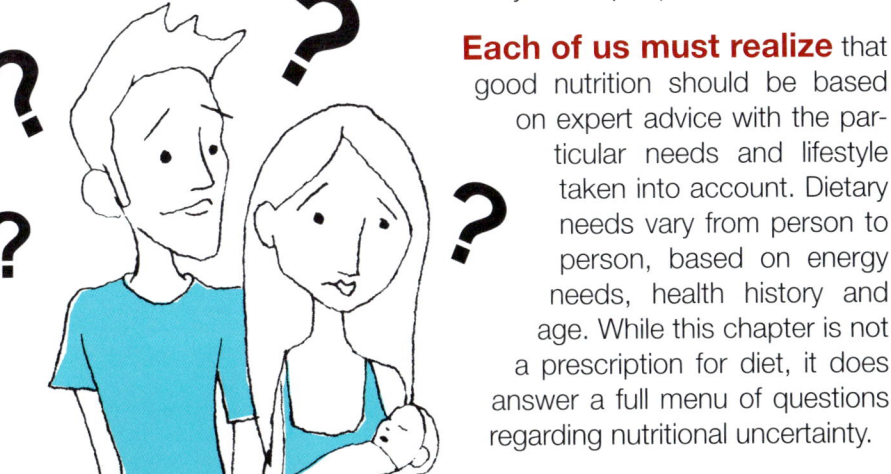

**Each of us must realize** that good nutrition should be based on expert advice with the particular needs and lifestyle taken into account. Dietary needs vary from person to person, based on energy needs, health history and age. While this chapter is not a prescription for diet, it does answer a full menu of questions regarding nutritional uncertainty.

# Q67 How Can the New Food Pyramid Help me?

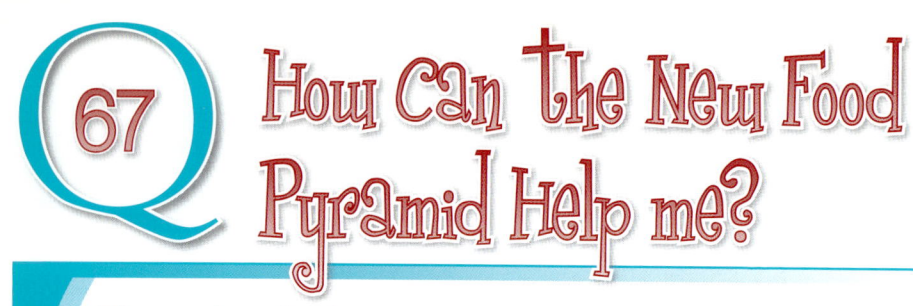

**The newly revised, user-friendly, color-coded** pyramid has taken a step in the right direction for all of us by making it EASY. The United States Department of Agriculture, (USDA) responded to the public who has become much more interested on fitness and health matters and demanded some direction on good nutrition.

It has been many years since the USDA first published the food pyramid we have all come to recognize. We refer to it time and time again. Dietitians can draw it and label it in their sleep. But since then, there has been one opinionated book after another claiming a better way—a better plan than the USDA pyramid.

The old pyramid was outdated. Life has changed in the last decade—people are more active and more stressed—some less active and more stressed. We are all getting fatter each year. If you really eat all the grains the old pyramid suggested, you might come to know how a cow feels grazing in the fields.

## The Newly Developed Food Pyramids

- Are color coded
- Are individualized based on age, gender and activity level
- Are no longer cookie-cutter with a one size fits all mentality
- Are accessible online

## *Color Coding*

- **Orange** for grains
- **Green** for vegetables
- **Red** for fruits
- **Blue** for dairy
- **Purple** for meat and beans
- **Yellow** for discretionary calories/oils

Color Coding makes it simple. There are six food categories. The revised pyramid tells you how much of each food group you should eat daily. The best part of the new pyramid is that fitness and nutrition experts are at long last partnering in their message that *exercise without proper nutrition or vice versa is not going to result in optimum health.* It is the essential combination of nutrition and physical activity that garners the most lifestyle benefits.

# Q68 What is the Bottom Line on Low-Carb Diets?

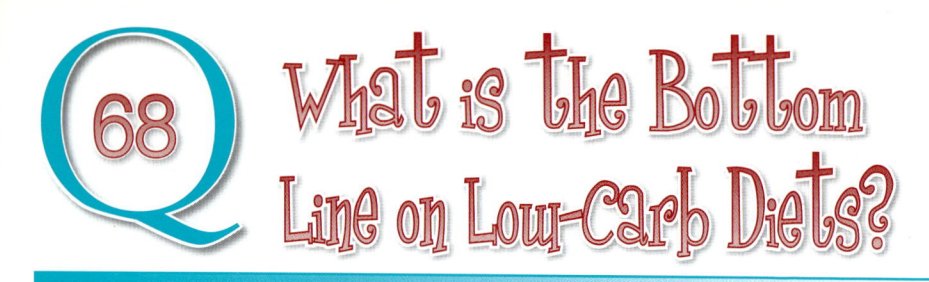

*We are carbophobic*—many perceive carbohydrates negatively with regard to nutrition. The **Low-Carb** diets have had their fifteen minutes of fame but it is over. For anyone still questioning the worth of carbohydrates…this is for you.

Most foods that aren't a fat or a protein are a carbohydrate. The trick is identifying which carbs are best. *Your brain and all your muscles require the glucose derived from carbs to keep you functioning. The majority of your vitamins and minerals come from this food group. Almost half or at least 40 per cent of your diet should come from carbohydrates but they should come from nutrient-rich fruit, vegetables and whole grains.*

There are essentially two types of carbohydrates—simple and complex. Both have a reason for being but if you want to lose weight… stay away from simple, processed carbs and eat complex ones.

## Bad Carbs-Simple and Processed

- Simple sugars
- Sweet white cereals
- White stuff like potatoes, rice and bread and bagels
- Alcohol
- Candy

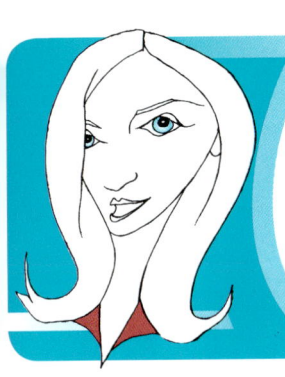

**CindySays...** *"The amount of calories you consume determines your weight—the kind of calories you consume determines your health!"*

- Soft drinks and sweet drinks
- Snack crackers and chips
- Cookies and cakes
- Pastries like doughnuts
- French fries
- Pizza
- Ice cream
- Most fast foods

## Good Carbs-Whole Grain and Nutrient Dense

- Whole grain breads
- Whole grain pastas
- Freshly prepared vegetables like broccoli and spinach
- Fresh fruits like apples, pears, berries, grapefruit
- Legumes and beans
- Brown rice
- Sweet potatoes

Remember, if you are trying to lose weight; plan to eat all food groups. *Eliminating a food group is never healthy or wise.* The bottom line which determines weight gain or weight loss is the amount of calories you consume compared to the amount of calories you expend. Partner with your best friend *(physical activity)* to manage your weight.

# Q69 How Do I Snack Healthfully?

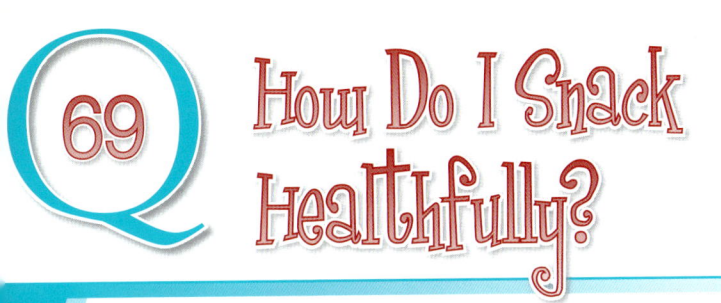

**Snacking is very beneficial and necessary for energy, metabolism and appetite control.** Eating processed carbs as a primary (daily) snack source, however, is a snacking disaster. The main culprits are regular and diet soft drinks, pretzels, cookies, crackers, animal crackers, candy bars, goldfish—vending machine carbs. Even though they may be low in calories, these snacks offer little in the way of good nutrition and create a craving for bad food that repeats itself. You should plan to eat 6 mini-meals a day rather than 3 large meals to keep your energy up and prevent undesirable food cravings.

## Think of Snacks as Mini Meals

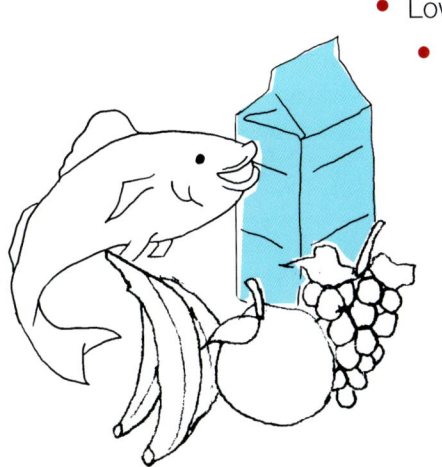

- Low-Fat Cottage Cheese
- Light yogurt
- Raw vegetables
- Raw unsalted almonds
- String cheese
- Low-fat dairy products
- Low sodium vegetable juice
- Dry roasted soy nuts
- Fresh fruit and berries

- Granola
- Pita pocket with tuna or salmon
- Baked sweet potato
- Whole grain wheat bagel with peanut butter
- Spreadable fruit on wheat toast
- Protein bar
- Lots and lots of water

# Q70 How Much Protein Do I Need Each Day?

**Basic nutrition is important to understand** as diet misconceptions will delay positive results. Designing meals to include the adequate amounts of protein as well as adequate amounts of carbohydrates and fats will help you reach health and fitness goals in the shortest amount of time.

**Unfortunately, we are served up a never ending "diet" buffet** with ample portions of confusion when reading about *high-protein diets, low-carb diets, and fat-free diets.* Protein is the topic of conversation in many health and fitness centers and while the Reference Daily Intake (RDI) has set a daily requirement, dieticians, nutritionists, fitness specialists, doctors and educators continue to debate the amount of protein we need daily.

## *What Does Protein Do For Us?*

- Provides energy
- Maintains muscles
- Repairs damaged cells
- Strengthens respiratory function
- Fortifies immune system
- Keeps hair skin and nails healthy

*This is an excellent reason to include lean protein in every meal!*

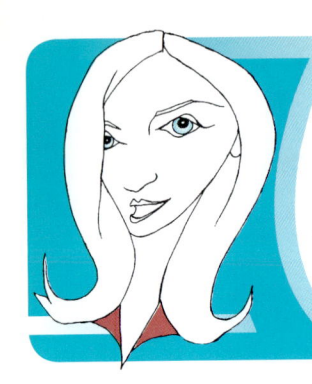

**CindySays**... *"While we probably don't need more than the RDI recommendation for protein to live, we may need more to thrive with our hectic lifestyles."*

*The Reference Daily Intake (RDI) is the daily dietary intake level of a nutrient considered sufficient to meet the requirements of nearly all (97–98%) healthy individuals in each life-stage and gender group. The RDI was formerly known as the Recommended Dietary Allowance (RDA). The RDI for protein is 0.8 grams of protein per kilogram of body weight. This recommendation has been found to be sufficient for most people.*

Because the RDI is based on satisfying minimum requirements to maintain basic function, some experts in the field of nutrition advocate higher protein needs for athletes performing endurance training and strength training. Research evidence suggests that sports athletes and serious weightlifters may require more than the RDI of protein in their diet to aid muscle growth and repair.

## What Part of Your Diet Should Be Made Up of Protein?

While the numbers listed above can be confusing, it might be simpler to break down your needs into what percentage of protein, carbohydrates and fats should make up your diet.

- *30% Protein*
- 40% Carbohydrates
- 30% Fat

## *Protein Can Facilitate Weight Loss?*

- Foods high in protein have great satiating power—*making you feel full and you stay satisfied longer because they empty from your stomach at a slower pace*
- High quality and lean sources of protein such as tuna, salmon, chicken, beef and eggs, prepared healthfully (low-fat) along with beans, legumes, fresh vegetables will facilitate healthy weight loss if *calories expended are more than calories ingested*
- Eat *fewer carbohydrates*, especially those that are highly processed

## *Stay Away From Poor Sources of Protein*

- Bacon
- Sausage
- Ground beef

## *Eat Good Sources of Protein*

- Skinless chicken breast
- Cooked lentils
- Tuna steak

A well-balanced diet along with regular exercise will give you the energy you need and the physique you desire. Plan to get the necessary protein and complex carbohydrates to support your active life.

# Q71 I Exercise Regularly— Am I Entitled to Dessert?

**I am a believer of everything in moderation—including moderation.** Saying goodbye to desserts and foods that you love would not be realistic or necessary.

**However, many who are make daily activity a priority do so with a built-in loophole.** Here's how it typically works. Rewards are given as a result of exercise. For instance, someone walks 2 miles—rewards themselves with a nice slice of cheesecake. Another takes a fitness class—goes to lunch and enjoys pie and ice cream after a salad. Still another who plays tennis for an hour—tips back a margarita and scoffs down a pile of tostado chips loaded with cheese and sour cream. They deserve it—they have earned it. In other words they see a healthy lifestyle as something of a hardship and therefore feel entitled to some sort of payback.

- The problem with this type of rational is these continual entitlements become habitual.
- Seeking restitution for every healthy lifestyle choice we make ultimately sabotages the progress we hope for.

Feeling entitled to a treat each time we sweat would be like skipping brushing after a good dental checkup…deciding not to buckle up because you've never had an accident…spending $100.00 impulsively because you saved 3 cents a gallon on gas.

Obviously, we don't want to live our life without appetizers, drinks or desserts or even impulse shopping. As I said, that is unnecessary and completely unrealistic not to mention boring.

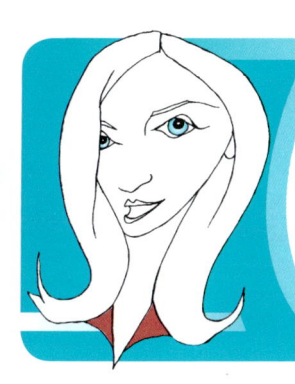

***CindySays**...*"Rewarding good habits with bad ones will always leave you with a deficit on the good habit side."*

Here is where the moderation comes in. Every now and then a food, a dessert or a treat is completely in order. How often and how much is the key issue.

## *Imagine Rewarding Good Habits With— Of All Things—GOOD HABITS!*

- After that walk reward yourself with a relaxing facial and a soothing soak in a tub.
- After the fitness class, reward yourself with a protein drink blended with fresh, delectable fruit.
- After the tennis game, reward yourself with…oh well, go ahead and have some chips and margaritas…let's not be ridiculous.

**Allow for some indulgences for your healthy choices.** You ARE entitled to a few. Try thinking of them as allowances instead of rights. And remember, healthy habits such as exercise, good food and relaxation are your friends, not your enemies. Embrace them and let them motivate you into adopting even more life enriching behaviors.

# Q72 How Do I Stop Overeating at Holiday Time?

**Three days after Thanksgiving, we sit in amazement** of our traditional celebratory feast. With leftovers from a whopping 27-pound turkey still hogging all the space in the refrigerator, we wonder how many more times we can re-warm and devour another calorie-laden plate of food. Just around the corner comes Hanukkah, Christmas and Kwanzaa. **Why do holidays sabotage our good intentions for better health?**

Holidays are open season for eating and drinking too much. The family traditions, open houses, spiritual celebrations, shopping excursions and office parties are just a few ways we find additional opportunities to consume excessive calories, fat, sweets and alcohol. Oftentimes, we have two to three events in a single day call it a success when we can juggle our schedules so that we hit every one of them. Of course, the idea of socializing draws us there, but take away the delectable culinary treats and beverages and you will find an empty room.

To make matters worse, during this hectic time, we often put exercise on the back burner to fit everything else in. This is the real problem—the deal breaker—which explains why we find ourselves crying in our champagne on New Years Eve. Yearly rituals bring us to the start of a new year with shame in our hearts and extra pounds on our hips—we then vow to give up everything we love and start all over again. We need a plan of action—ACTION being the key word. *Expect to face abundance.*

## Take a Proactive Approach

- Decide to attend the functions with more discretion
- Be selective when it comes to food and cocktails
- Be mindful of portion control
- Eat a healthy snack and drink a glass of water before each social gathering
- Avoid making a beeline to the bar or food table
- Give yourself a little time to socialize

## Beverages

- Normally have three drinks?—Reduce that number
- Substitute healthier alcohol-free beverages
- Try sparkling water with lime in a champagne flute

## Food

- Only sample a few hors d'oeuvres that are new or interesting
- Fill in with healthy choices—fresh fruits and veggies minus high calories dips
- Choose one dessert and enjoy it instead of having a bite of all of them

## Exercise

- Make physical activity a priority in the midst of juggling a lively social calendar
- Avoid freeing up time for holiday functions at the expense of your workouts

- Activity is your body's greatest stress reliever so recognize its value
- Maximize your workouts by cutting all socialization time in the gym

**Finally, when it is time to prepare your own holiday meals,** give yourself permission to deviate slightly from traditional high calorie offerings to include a few healthier options. Try using some low fat ingredients in your cooking and understand that not everything you serve tastes better with gravy or sauce on it.

Now this friendly fitness advice is not given to put a damper on your holiday fun—it simply asks you to do a little planning in order for you to move through the holidays with more energy and less guilt. Take what suggestions you can live with and toss the rest over your shoulder.

# Q73 I Love Buffets—How Can I Avoid Them?

**All you can eat buffets can be detrimental to a weight loss plan** but it is unrealistic to expect you to never visit one again.

**Everyone has been there and done it.** You take a plate and walk through the beautiful buffet line and take a little of this and a little of that. Well, who are we kidding? A little of thirty or more food choices is a mountain of food!

**But we've all had the occasional going-away buffet luncheon** for a co-worker or business travel that leaves us with limited choices in restaurants. If you have ever vacationed in Las Vegas, you'll have more luck at the black jack table than you will avoiding at least one trip to a tempting buffet. Cruises offer all-day, all-night buffets which seem to excite people more than the ports of call. It seems inevitable that we are going to attend our share of calorie laden buffets.

The key consideration lies in *food selection and portion size*. The most common mistake is to arrive at the buffet table so hungry that anything and everything finds its way onto your plate. It is like going to the grocery store on an empty stomach. You find it impossible to stick to your shopping list and end up buying items that are not healthy choices.

*Eat something light an hour before with a glass of water and...*

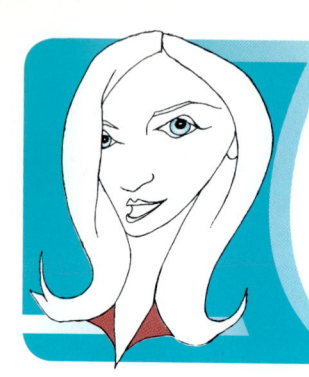

***CindySays***...*"It is not a race to see how many trips a person can make to the buffet."*

## *Choose Well*

- Lean cuts of meat and fish—avoid breaded and fried
- Fresh or grilled vegetables—avoid ones covered with sauces
- Go easy on the salad—use small amounts of light dressings—no croutons!
- Small portions of a select number of foods

***It takes your brain 15 to 20 minutes to get the signal that your stomach is satisfied so...***

## *Eat Slow*

- Sip on your beverage and allow yourself to get the signal
- If you go back for seconds—choose healthy foods such as fresh fruits
- Remember getting "your money's worth" at buffets can add another 7000 calories
- Fight the urge to gorge

# Q74 How Do I Avoid Gaining Weight in College?

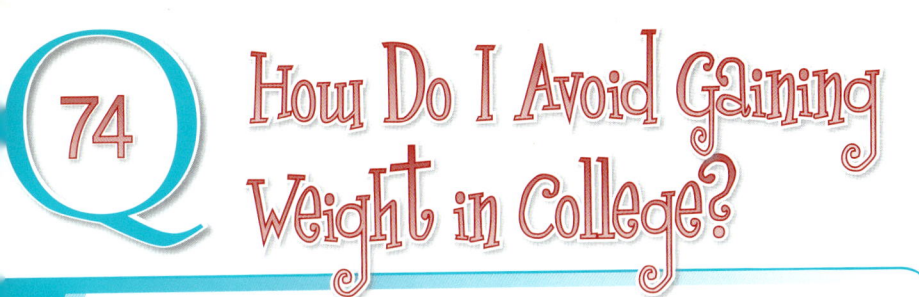

Awareness about anything is power. **The freshman fifteen** is slang assigned to the common weight gain by men and women during the first year of college. Wow—not an appealing thought to most students. But, it is not inevitable. In fact, while many do gain, some actually manage to lose or maintain their current weight.

**Considering the major changes that occur** in a new student's life, it's easy to appreciate some physical consequences. After all, it can be one of the most difficult years in life. Living arrangements change—family and friends are left behind—responsibility increases—and then college life offers a freedom like never before.

## *What Causes the Weight Gain?*

- College meal plans make food accessible day and night in dining halls
- Foods, including desserts, are served up "all you can eat" buffet-style
- In an attempt to accommodate a variety of tastes and nutrition needs of a diverse student body, a wide array of foods are offered
- Fast foods are prevalent in college settings
- Late night eating is a common occurrence
- Studying often includes snacking

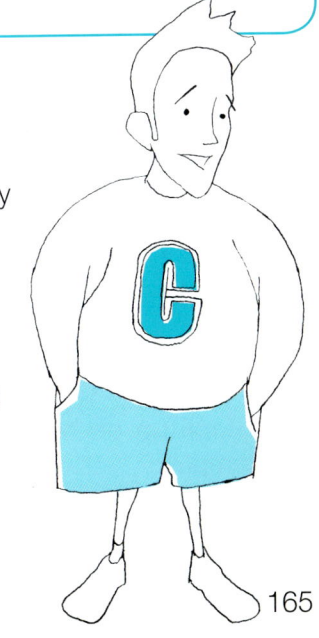

- Social gatherings always include high calorie foods such as pizza, chips, wings, creamy lattes and sodas
- Alcohol (loaded with empty calories) is accessible
- Well-meaning relatives send high-calorie goody baskets
- Lots of snack machines filled with unhealthy choices
- Normal exercise routines are disrupted or eliminated
- Sleep habits vary day to day
- Parties, parties and more parties—oh and don't forget after-parties

Of course, when you factor in freshman freedom to the list above it sometimes adds up to 15 pounds of freshman fat. But, don't despair, there are some lessons to be learned here that can help you defy the odds. Believe it or not, in addition to the academics there are some other wonderful things college life offers.

The beauty of being on your own at school is the way it persuades you to take charge of your life. You learn that you need to manage not only your money and your time but also—your health. If you realize this when you arrive on campus, you will be less likely to fall into the food traps.

## Keep These Tips in Mind

- Plan to eat three times a day, making healthful choices at the buffet rather than trying everything
- Avoid desserts most days or limit them to "just a taste"
- Watch the size of the portions you put on your plate and be careful about seconds
- Stock up on healthful snacks so that vending machines won't be tempting
- Just say NO to the alcohol—freshmen usually aren't 21 so it is illegal AND fattening

- Ask that parents send things like protein bars and bottled water rather than home baked cookies
- Don't skip meals — intense hunger leads to poor choices
- Eat a healthful meal before going to party so you will make better choices and consume less of the high-fat foods
- Find ways and places to exercise
- Take a daily multi-vitamin
- Drink plenty of water and avoid the sodas
- Partying can be good — Dance, dance, dance

## *Your Activity Level is the Key to Weight Management*

- If you're eating smart but failing to exercising, the pounds will find you
- Most colleges have a fitness facility membership included in the tuition — use it
- Walk as much as possible and always take the stairs
- Join an intramural team for exercise and to meet like-minded friends
- Schedule a physical education class whenever possible
- If going to classes involves riding a bus or tram, consider riding a bicycle

It is important also to keep in mind that some weight gain is natural. Most first-year college students are still growing and their bone density should be increasing. Make it a priority to see your physician regularly for a complete physical. Good health involves far more than knowing how much you weigh. Most importantly — enjoy the best college has to offer and don't fret over **the freshman fifteen!** College will enlighten you in many ways — pay attention to what it teaches you about managing your health.

# Q75 What Should I Eat After a Workout?

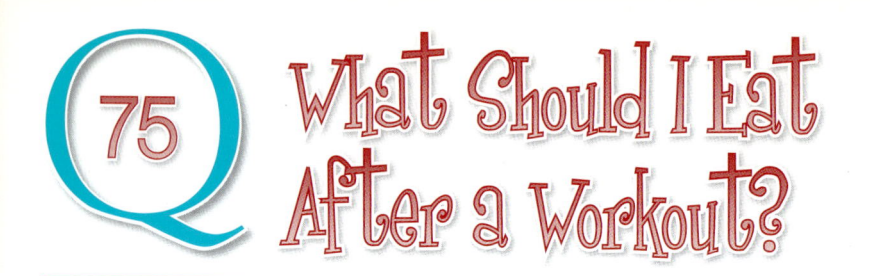

**Optimum recovery with regard to nutrition and hydration** should be thought of as part of your training. Attending to these needs immediately following your workout will greatly enhance your ability to perform with your best possible effort the next day.

## If You Exercise Less Than 60 Minutes at a Time

**WATER** is the body's number one need before, during and after exercise. Dehydration, particularly in heat and humidity, is the greatest potential risk facing active people today. Exercising out of doors makes adequate hydration more of an issue than exercising indoors where there is usually less heat and humidity.

## If You Exercise Longer Than One Hour

**WATER plus CARBOHYDRATES and PROTEIN** needs to be replenished *especially if it is an intense pace.* Endurance workouts break down muscle tissue and deplete energy. Energy that comes from the muscle is known as glycogen. This is where the carbohydrates and protein come into the picture. Consuming carbohydrates and protein soon after exercising has stopped promotes muscle recover and replenishes the glycogen lost during physical exertion.

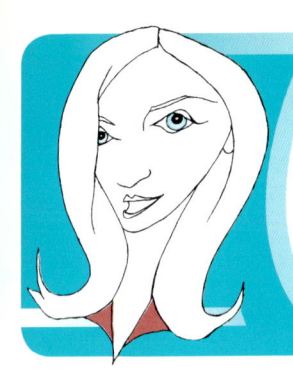

*CindySays...* "How and when we fuel our bodies is important. It requires a little pre-planning but the payoff is great!

## What's the Best Way to Do This?

**A CARBOHYDRATE and PROTEIN RATIO of 3:1** (3 grams of carbohydrates to 1 gram of protein) after exercise is best. A liquid such as skim milk or a shake is a great way to do this as it is quickly digested. Skim milk contains a great deal of water in it which helps replace lost fluids from sweating and both carbohydrates and protein.

## *EXAMPLES*

- Fruit and low fat cheese
- Sports drink and dry roasted soy nuts
- Turkey breast on whole wheat bagel
- Yogurt with fruit such as a banana
- Tuna and tomato on wheat toast
- Vegetable bean soup and whole wheat roll
- Low fat cottage cheese and fresh fruit
- Melted low fat cheese on whole grain English muffin and orange
- Rice cakes with peanut butter spread and fruit juice or sports drink
- Protein shake made with yogurt and fresh fruit

## Q76 How Do I Keep my Child from Snacking?

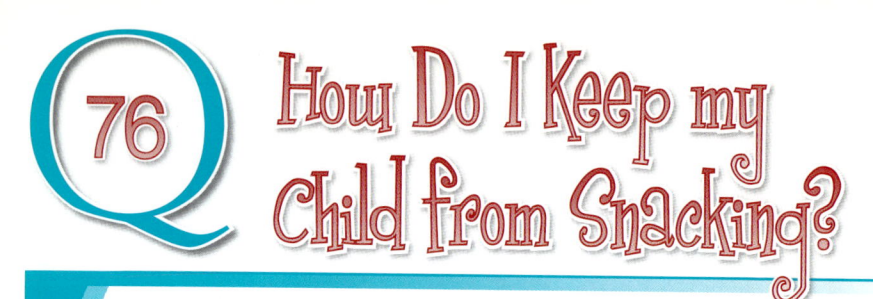

**You shouldn't. Don't ban—plan!** Snacking is a *healthy habit* for children to get into if planned properly. An important consideration is the quality of snacks you give them. Think of snacking as an opportunity to add appealing nutrition to your child's diet. It will keep their energy level constant, their body functioning efficiently, and prevent them from becoming overly hungry. The hungrier they are, the poorer their food choices become.

Enjoy this time with your children by having a light snack with them. Eating 4 to 6 small meals a day rather than three large meals is beneficial for adults too!

### Healthy Snacks to Keep in Your Kitchen

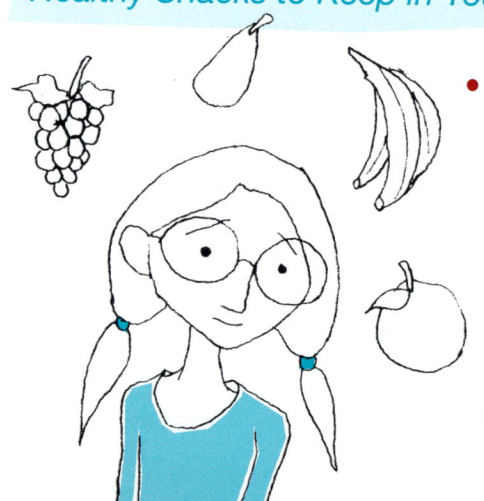

- Fresh fruits
- Bite-sized vegetables
- Yogurt
- Almonds
- Raisons and other dried fruits
- Whole wheat breads
- Low fat milk
- String cheese

# Q77 What's the Quickest Diet Fix?

**Stop drinking your calories!** Fruit juices, coffee drinks and sodas are liquid calories that don't make you feel satisfied for very long. Eliminating these nutritionally empty calories will go a long way toward a healthier body and weight loss. Instead, opt for low or no-calorie beverages like water, tea and skim milk that offer some nutritional benefit.

## Best to Worst

- Water-*This should be your main hydration beverage*
- Unsweetened tea
- Low-fat or skim milk
- 100% fruit juice with no sugar added
- Non-calorie sweetened-*This should be consumed sparingly*

# 78 Q What Does Low-Glycemic and High-Glycemic Mean?

**Not all carbohydrate foods are created equal;** in fact they behave quite differently once we ingest them into our bodies. The Glycemic Index predicts how quickly a carbohydrate causes blood sugar—*glucose*— to rise. Foods with refined sugars and simple starches, like candy and white bread, generally have a high glycemic index, while high fiber foods made up of complex carbohydrates, such as whole grains and vegetables, have a low glycemic index.

**The Glycemic Index or GI** distinguishes the difference by ranking carbohydrates—*and assigning them a number*—according to the way they affect blood glucose levels. Low GI carbs only produce small fluctuations in blood glucose and insulin levels and are the carbs we should be eating. Certain carbs and beverages trigger an undesirable insulin response. These are labeled High-Glycemic and should be avoided.

## *Eat Mainly Low GI Carbs for Better Health*

- Releases glucose slowly into the blood stream
- Balances energy levels
- Makes you feel fuller for longer periods of time
- Decreases blood cholesterol levels
- Reduces risk of heart disease and diabetes
- Aids in weight loss
- Diminishes hunger

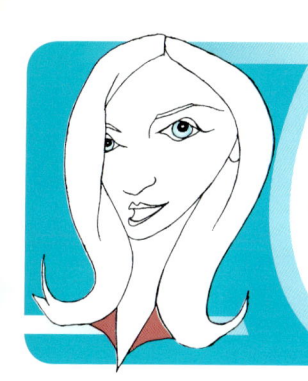

*CindySays...* "*For good health and successful weight management eat more Lower GI foods and less High GI foods!*"

## Learn the Difference

- **Low GI**—*Less than 55*
  - Sour dough bread 54
  - Apple juice 40
  - Pumpernickel 50
  - Oatmeal 48
  - Pasta 54

- **Intermediate GI**—*56 to 69*
  - Croissant 67
  - Soft-drinks 63
  - Raisin bran 61
  - Whole wheat bread 65

- **High GI**—*More than 70*
  - White bread 70
  - Corn flakes 80
  - Doughnut 76
  - White rice 98

## Choose Wisely With These Simple Tips

- Select food primarily on overall nutrition such as their vitamin, mineral and fiber content
- Try to include at least one low GI food with each meal
- Limit your processed, refined, starchy foods
- Eat whole grain, pumpernickel and oat bran bread rather than white bread
- Enjoy the variety of at least five servings of fresh fruit and vegetables a day
- Choose brown rice more often than instant rice and yams instead of white and/or instant potatoes
- Monitor your portion sizes—larger portions raise blood glucose more dramatically
- Eat five to six small meals a day to manage your appetite

## Chapter 7

# FINAL THOUGHTS

**We all face physical and emotional challenges** in our hectic worlds. Some seem insurmountable at times but I believe a strong body is capable of withstanding much more than a weak one—there is wisdom in the old adages, "survival of the fittest" and "only the strong survive."

**In today's competitive environment,** acquiring a strong physical self and striving to strike a balance in our lifestyle choices can put us on the path toward better health. We should all be mindful and in control of the amount of time we work as opposed to play; the amount of time we are active as opposed to sedentary; the amount of nutritious foods we consume as opposed to the amount of foods made up of empty calories; and the amount of time we are interacting with people as opposed to time that is quiet and contemplative.

**We must be interested in improving our own physicality.** Managing our time to allow regular activity is never wasteful. The process of working out is packed with gratifying moments which are palpable and measurable. With every step, every push-up, every pound, every breath, we gain power—not only physically, but emotionally as well.

Value your body—listen intently to its needs. They are simple—good food, appropriate activity, a positive environment and adequate rest. Fill your life with these and you will find health and abundant happiness in your hectic world.

# How Do I Stick With my Healthy Lifestyle?

**Surveys show that approximately 90 percent** of people who attempt lifestyle changes totally abandon them after only 17 days.

Wow—not very encouraging now is it? Almost makes you want to rethink this whole changing your life thing! Wanting to adopt a healthy lifestyle for the long haul is a noble idea and certainly a lofty goal. But, most of us think in terms of giving things up when we come face to face with our own mortality. Instead, I believe we should think in terms of adding to our life.

## Why We Continue to Fail

- We set unrealistic goals and expectations
- We attempt to make drastic lifestyle habits
- We abandon our goals at the first sign of failure
- We feel deprived and uncomfortable

I was just like many who make resolutions in life with a strong desire to change. But, when I looked pragmatically into why I was failing in these attempts, two things just didn't add up.

*I was biting off more than I could chew*
*I didn't like giving up everything I liked*

## Failure

The truth is we don't like giving things up — in fact we hate it. If all we see ourselves doing in our quest for better health is *GIVING UP* things, why is it such a surprise that we end up *GIVING UP?*

Why not go at it backwards? Why not, instead of giving up -- we start *ADDING TO?* Yes, that is what I said -- start adding things to your life. We all deserve some of the good things in this world. It is my sincere belief that deprivation ultimately leads to rejection.

I trust if we *add enough good things* to our life and *put enough good things* in our mouths, we will naturally want *less of the bad things.* It is a simple philosophy but it has worked for me and it is a plan you can most assuredly stick to.

### It Goes Something Like This

- **Concerned about eating too many fats?** Start adding 5 fruits or vegetables to your daily meals. My bet is, once you've added these you won't be quite as hungry for the fats.

- **Finding that you consume too much junk food?** Try a protein bar or a fiber bar and a cup of warm tea at those times when you would otherwise have a candy bar and a soft drink.

- **Discovering that you mindlessly munch when you are not even hungry** but rather anxious or upset? Give yourself a stress break and find a quiet place where you can calm your spirit and breathe deeply.

- **Thinking of going shopping for something new?** Try a yoga mat and video for a new invigorating experience; a balance ball to sit on at your desk or to use at home to strengthen your abs and back; a pedometer so that you can see just how many steps you take in a day and so you can aim for a few more steps each day.

- **Looking for a shortcut to building a better body** through harmful diet and weight loss pills? Pop a multivitamin once a day for genuine health.

- **Feeling overcome with nervous energy and need a smoke?** Put on some walking shoes and use that energy to give yourself a stronger heart and lungs not to mention a new lease on life.

- **Longing for that drink to make you feel better?** Make it water— the real fountain of youth.

- **Eager to get home from work to find your favorite spot on the couch?** Try turning on wonderful music that makes you want to move and dance—even if it is a slow dance.

- **Struggling to fall asleep** and want to sneak to the kitchen for a late night snack? Try opening a book that interests you and takes you further than your kitchen.

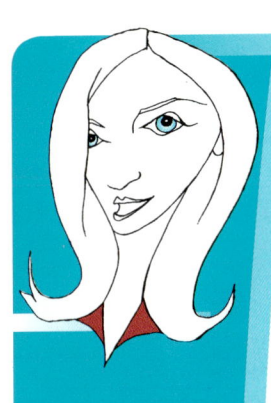

## *CindySays*...

- *Resolve to change only one or two unhealthy habits within a reasonable time frame.*

- *Set small goals based on your own wishes and desires. A resolution is sure to fail if it is not from your heart.*

- *Write down your plan of action to track your success and place it so that you see it often. Somehow, seeing it in black and white strengthens the conviction.*

- *Enlist the support of someone who can strengthen your motivation and to whom you can be accountable. Don't forget to do the same for him or her.*

- *Reward yourself when steps in the right direction are taken.*

- *Plan for the fact that you are going to have setbacks and be ready to jump right back onto the right track.*

# Valuable Insight from my Mentors

**We all have the ability to change our lives.** It can be exhilarating to liberate ourselves from old ways and try something new. But, it also can be frightening. When we desire change and improvement, we must accept there will be pitfalls and roadblocks along our path. Real change is not easy or simple—if fact, changing our mindset is usually the most remarkable change we have to make. For me, the times I sought advice were when I was most challenged and ready to throw in the towel. Sometimes from friends or family but most often from those who had faced far greater challenges than me. It was these people that would ultimately spark my desire to continue on or to stay the course. **Here are a few words of wisdom that I would like to share with you.**

*I've been absolutely terrified every moment of my life and I've never let it keep me from doing a single thing I wanted to do* — Georgia O'Keefe

Oftentimes, we hesitate to start an exercise program or take the first step because we fear the unknown.

- I'm going to look silly
- I just know it will hurt
- This will probably be a big waste of money
- I have no idea what to wear
- I don't really believe it will work

Inactivity and dwelling on fear of the unknown is extremely detrimental to your mind and body. Going outside your home and taking a brisk walk in the sunshine and crisp air can change your perspective immediately and boost your immunity. It's OK if that first step is a leap of faith. Believe you can do more and life will reward you.

*Life is not a stress rehearsal* — Loretta Laroche

Finding ourselves entwined in what might happen prevents us from being free to see what is happening. Living your life in the moment is so much more pleasant than worrying about what might come next. Open your eyes and look for possibility.

- Pick up a Pilates video to try at home
- Volunteer at an assisted living home or nearby grade school
- Enroll in a dance class
- Sign up for bowling lessons
- Learn to swim or help others learn to swim
- Vow to try a new activity each month

*The greatest gift that you can give yourself is a little bit of your own attention* —
Anthony J. DeAngelo

Give generously to yourself. Taking care of yourself is integral to taking care of your loved ones. If you don't value yourself, no one else will value you.

- Take a multi-vitamin every day
- Drink plenty of water and get adequate rest
- Try yoga, tai chi or anything that includes breath control and relaxation

# Glossary

## Get to Know Your Health and Fitness Terms

## A

### Abs
Abbreviation for abdominal muscles.

### Absolute Strength
The maximum amount a person can lift in one repetition.

### Acquired Aging
The acquisition of characteristics commonly associated with aging but that are, in fact, caused by immobility or sedentary living.

### Active Stretch
Muscles are stretched using the contraction of the opposing muscle, (antagonist). For an example stretching the triceps, requires the biceps to contract.

### Aerobic Exercise
Activity in which the body is able to supply adequate oxygen to the working muscles, for a period of time. Running, cross-country skiing and cycling are examples of aerobic activities.

### Anabolic Steroid
Synthetic chemical that mimics the muscle building characteristics of the male hormone testosterone.

### Anaerobic Exercise
Activity in which oxygen demands of muscles are so high that they rely upon an internal metabolic process for oxygen, resulting in lactic acid build up. Short bursts of "all-out" activities such as sprinting or weightlifting are anaerobic.

### Anaerobic Threshold
The point at which you begin working your muscles without oxygen, from an aerobic level, believed to be at about 87% of your Maximum Heart Rate.

### Asanas
Various yoga poses.

### Atrophy
Decrease in size and functional ability—withering away of muscle tissue or organs.

# B

### Ballistic Stretch
A more vigorous stretch by using a swinging or bouncing motion.

### Barbell
Weight used for exercise, consisting of a rigid handle 5-7 feet long, with detachable metal discs at each end.

### Basal Metabolic Rate or BMR
The number of calories your body burns at rest to maintain normal body functions.

### Bodybuilding
Weight training that changes physical appearance.

### Body Composition
The breakdown of your body make-up—for example your fat, lean muscle, bone and water content.

### Bone Density
Soundness of the bones within the body, low density can be a result of osteoporosis.

# C

### Carbohydrate
Compounds that contain carbon, hydrogen and oxygen used by the body as a fuel source.

### Cholesterol
A fat lipid which has both good and bad implications within the human body. Good being known as HDL and bad being LDL. A high LDL is associated with heart disease and stroke. A high HDL is desirable and can be improved by physical exercise.

### Chronic Disease
A disease or illness that is associated with lifestyle or environment factors as opposed to infectious diseases.

### Circuit Training
Going quickly from one exercise apparatus to another and doing a prescribed number of exercises or time on each apparatus. This keeps pulse rate high and promotes overall fitness by generally working all muscle groups as well as heart and lungs.

### Cross-training
Integrating variety of different activities into your regular workout routine to avoid overuse injuries and to prevent boredom. Performing cycling, running and weight-training is an example of cross-training.

### Crunches
A type of exercise which promotes abdominal strength.

# D

### Deficiency
A less than optimal level of either one or more nutrients, often resulting in poor health.

### Dehydration
Excessive fluid loss from the body, caused by perspiration, urination, evaporation or illness.

### Delts
Abbreviation for deltoids—the large triangular muscles of the shoulder which raise the arm away from the body.

### DOMS or Delayed Onset Muscle Soreness
A condition sometimes felt after exercise, especially if it is weight orientated or intense. Caused by the very small tears within a muscle which generally lasts for 24 to 72 hours.

### Dumbbell
Weights attached to a short bar that can be held in one hand and are often used in pairs.

# E

### Endurance
Ability of a muscle to produce force continually over a period of time.

### Extension
Describes a body part, for example your hand, neck, leg or trunk, going from a bent to a straight position.

# F

### Fat
Often referred to as lipids, or triglycerides, one of the main food groups, containing nine calories per gram.

### Fatigue
Weariness or exhaustion resulting from exertion.

*Flex*
To bend or decrease angle of a joint.

*Flexibility*
Range of movement in a joint or group of joints.

*Free Weights*
Weights which are not attached to a machine or driven by cables or chains. Barbells and dumbbells are examples of free weights.

# G

*Gluteals or Glutes*
Abbreviation for gluteus or buttock muscles.

*Glycemic Index or GI*
A system that measures the extent to which various foods raise the blood sugar level. The benchmark is white bread, which has a GI of 100. The higher the score, the greater the extents of blood sugar raise.

*Glycogen*
The form in which carbohydrates take when stored in the muscles.

# H

*Hamstrings*
The group of three muscles on the back of your thighs that connect from the lower part of the pelvis to just below the knees. They allow you to bend your knees and straighten your legs at the hips.

*Hypertension*
High blood pressure.

*Hypertrophy*
Increase in size of muscle fiber.

# I

### *Internal Obliques*
Muscles that run upward and inward from the hip bones to the lower ribs, allowing you to rotate and bend at the waist.

### *Intervals*
Speed workouts, usually run on a track, with short distances at a specific pace interspersed with rest periods of slower running or walking.

### *Isometric Exercise*
Muscular contraction where muscle maintains a constant length and joints do not move. These exercises are usually performed against a wall or other immovable object.

### *Isotonic Exercise*
Muscular action in which there is a change in length of muscle and weight, keeping tension constant. Lifting free weights is a classic isotonic exercise.

# L

### *Lactic Acid*
A by-product of anaerobic—high-intensity—exercise that collects in the muscle and causes fatigue.

### *Lats*
Abbreviation for Latissimus dorsi—large muscles of the back that move the arms downward, backward and internally rotate.

### *Lean Body Mass*
Everything in the body except for fat, including bone, organs, skin, nails and all body tissue including muscle.

### *Lifestyle*
Individual patterns of your typical life.

### Ligament
A flexible, non-elastic tissue that connects bone to bone.

### Lumbar
Lower region of you spine, vertebrates L1 to L5. Used for bending and extending the body forward and back.

# M

### Maximum Heart Rate or MHR
Theoretical maximum heart rate one can achieve during his or her greatest effort in exercise.

### Metabolism
The sum total of the chemical reactions in the body at rest or during exercise.

### Muscle
Tissue consisting of fibers organized into bands or bundles that contract to cause bodily movement.

### Muscularity
Another term for definition, indicating fully delineated muscles and absence of fat.

# O

### Obliques
Abbreviation for external obliques which are the muscles to either side of abdominals that rotate and flex the trunk.

### Osteoporosis
A progressive condition more commonly found in older women characterized by decrease in bone mass with decreased density and enlargement of bone spaces producing porosity and fragility.

### Overload Principle
Applying a greater load than normal to a muscle to increase its capability.

# P

## Perceived Exertion
The level of intensity you feel your body is exerting during exercise on a scale of 6 to 20. An unscientific way of monitoring and staying within a safe heart rate range.

## Plyometrics
Exercises designed to generate the greatest amount of force in the shortest amount of time.

## Power
Strength combined with speed.

## Power Training
System of weight training using low repetitions and heavy weight.

## Progressive Resistance
A training method where weight is increased as muscles gain strength and endurance.

# Q

## Quads
Abbreviation for quadriceps muscles—muscles of the front portion of the upper legs.

# R

## ROM or Range of Motion
Range of motion often used to assess a person's flexibility in a joint.

## Rectus Abdominis
The muscle extending the entire length of the abdomen, from the lower three ribs to the top of the pubic bone that enable you to stand upright and bend at the waist.

### Repetition or Rep
A single movement, as in doing one push-up. This is going down and then going back up. There are typically 8 to 12 reps in a set.

### Resting Heart Rate
Heart rate measure taken during complete rest.

### Rhomboids
The muscles that pull your shoulder blades inward.

### R.I.C.E. or Rest Ice Compression Elevation
The formula for treating an injury such as a strain or sprain.

## S

### Set
A number of repetitions of a specific strength training exercise. For example, a set will contain several repetitions.

### Shin Splints
The generic term for pain in the front portion of the lower leg. Most often caused by inflammation of the tendons which can result when they are subjected to too much force for too long.

### Sprain
An injury to the ligament.

### Static Stretch
A simple muscle stretch that goes just to the point of gentle tension and is held steadily for several seconds without moving or bouncing.

### Strain
An injury to the tendon or muscle.

### Stretch Reflex
A protective, involuntary nerve reaction that causes muscles to contract. Bouncing or overstretching can trigger the reflex in which muscles are trying to protect themselves from damage.

# T

### Target Heart Rate or THR
The ideal intensity level at which your heart is being exercised but not overworked. Determined by taking a percentage of your maximum heart rate.

### Target Heart Rate Range or THRR
The heart rate range determined by the American College of Sports Medicine to be optimum for improving aerobic fitness.

### Tendon
A flexible, non-elastic tissue that connects muscle to bone.

### Trapezius or Traps
The triangular muscles stretching across your back from the spine to the shoulder blades and collarbone.

### Triceps
The muscles on the back of the upper arms that straighten your elbows and allow you to push your arms forward.

# W

### Weight-bearing Exercise
Exercise in which you support your weight or lift weight. Lifting weights or doing weight-bearing exercise (such as running or walking) can help slow the rate of bone loss and therefore reduce fractures.

# Y

### Yoga
A system of exercise for acquiring strength, flexibility and which facilitates relaxation.

To order additional copies of
**CindySays®... "You Can Find Health in Your Hectic World"**

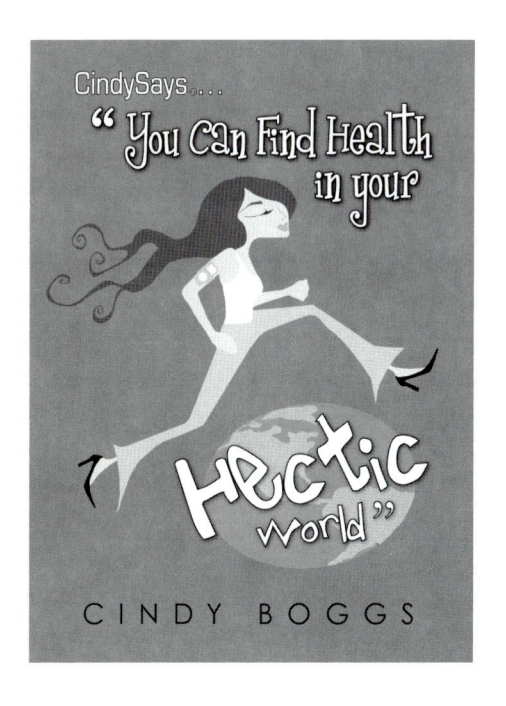

Visit
**www.cindysays.com**